Traditional Chinese Cosmetic Therapy

Chief-Editor: Zhao Xin Li Guohua

Academy Press [Xue Yuan]

First Edition 1998
ISBN7 – 5077 – 0358 – 4

Traditional Chinese Cosmetic Therapy
Chief – Editor: Zhao Xin   Li Guohua
Published by
Academy Press [Xue Yuan]
11 Wanshoulu Xijie, Beijing 100036, China

Distributed by
China International Book Trading Corporation
35 Chegongzhuang Xilu, Beijing 100044, China
P. O. Box 399, Beijing, China

Printed in the People's Republic of China

Preface

Traditional Chinese Medicine and Pharmacology(TCMP) has a long history. It summed up abundant clinical experience in the struggle against diseases. It has formed an integrated, unique and first of all, a scientific system of both theory and clinical practice. On the fundamental principle of 'Zhengtiguannian' (Wholism) and 'Bianzhenglunzhi' (Treatment of the same disease with different therapies). TCM treatment is effective for various kinds of diseases with few side-effect taken. At present, a great upsurge in learning, practising and studying TCM is just in the ascendant. For the benefit of people of all countries, we compiled this series of 'Collections of Traditional Chinese Medicine' in order to promote the spread of traditional Chinese medicine all over the world.

In this book, we introduced comprehensively traditional Chinese cosmetic therapies. This book is the best for those foreign friends who want to learn and master traditional Chinese medicine.

May everyone of all nations enjoy a healthy life!

Chief − Editor

Contents

Part One   Treatment for Diseases
   Chapter One   Ephelis ··· (1)
   Chapter Two   Moth-Patch ··· (5)
   Chapter Three   Acne ·· (8)
   Chapter Four   Wart ·· (17)
   Chapter Five   Peripheral Facial Paralysis ································· (21)
   Chapter Six   Thyroid Adenoma ·· (27)
   Chapter Seven   Calvities ·· (31)
   Chapter Eight   Simple Obesity ··· (38)
   Chapter Nine   Bromhidrosis ·· (50)
   Chapter Ten   Seborrheic Dermatitis ··· (54)
   Chapter Eleven   Xerosis Pilorum ··· (57)
   Chapter Twelve   Achromotrichia ··· (60)
   Chapter Thirteen   Halitosis ·· (67)
   Chapter Fourteen   Hygiene of Oral Cavity ······································ (71)
   Chapter Fifteen   Chilblain ·· (78)

Part Two   Commonly Used Drugs
   Radix Ginseng ·· (83)
   Radix et Rhizoma Rhei ··· (86)
   Rhizoma Dioscoreae ··· (88)
   Fructus Corni ··· (90)
   Rhizoma Ligustici Chuanxiong ·· (92)
   Fructus Ligustri Lucidi ·· (95)
   Radix Polygoni Multiflori ··· (96)
   Radix Asparagi ·· (100)
   Radix Salviae Miltiorrhizae ··· (101)
   Radix Astragali seu Hedysari ··· (103)
   Radix Angelicae Sinensis ··· (107)
   Semen Coicis ·· (111)
   Cortex Lycii Radicis ··· (113)
   Radix Rehmanniae ··· (117)
   Radix Rehmanniae Praeparata ··· (117)
   Herba Asari ··· (123)
   Fructus Lycii ·· (127)
   Semen Persicae ··· (129)

Part Three Commonly Used Prescriptions

Anti-inflammatory and Analgesic Bolus ······················ (132)
Anti-inflammatory Pill ······················ (133)
Acanthopanax Infusion ······················ (134)
Banlong Pill ······················ (135)
Baolong Pill ······················ (136)
Bolus for Activating Meridians ······················ (137)
Bolus for Severe Endogenous Wind-Syndrome ······················ (139)
Bolus of Arisaematis ······················ (140)
Bolus of Placenta Hominis ······················ (142)
Bolus of Precious Drugs ······················ (144)
Bolus of Storax ······················ (145)
Brain-Invigorating and Kidney-Tonifying Pill ······················ (147)
Cardiotonic Pill ······················ (148)
Decoction for Activating Blood Circulation ······················ (149)
Decoction for Eliminating Dampness and Relieving Rheumatism ······················ (151)
Decoction for Hemiplegia ······················ (152)
Decoction for Invigorating Spleen and
Nourishing heart ······················ (153)
Decoction for Invigorating Yang ······················ (155)
Decoction for Mild Hemiplegia ······················ (156)
Decoction for Removing Blood Stasis in the Chest ······················ (158)
Decoction for Sterility ······················ (160)
Decoction for Treating Rheumatism ······················ (161)
Decoction of Bupleuri Adding Os Draconis
and Concha Ostreae ······················ (163)
Decoction of Bupleuri and Puerariae for
Expelling Evil from Muslces ······················ (165)
Decoction of Cimicifugae and
Astragali seu Hedysari ······················ (166)
Decoction of Cinnamomi Aconiti ······················ (168)
Decoction of Cinnamomi, Glycyrrhizae, etc. ······················ (169)
Decoction of Cinnamomi, Paeoniae and Aemarrhenae ······················ (170)
Antipyretic and Antitoxic Bolus ······················ (172)
Bolus of Calculus Bovis for Purging the Heart-Fire ······················ (173)
Bolus of Citri Grandis ······················ (173)
Bolus of Rhei and Eupolyphaga seu Steleophaga ······················ (175)
Bolus of Six Drugs Including Rehmannia ······················ (177)
Bolus of Ten Powerful Tonics ······················ (179)
Cow-bezoar Bolus for Clearing Away Heat
of the Upper Part of the Body ······················ (180)
Decoction for Clearing Away Pestilent
Factors and Detoxification ······················ (181)
Decoction for Clearing Heat in Ying System ······················ (183)
Decoction for Strngthening Middle

Jiao and Benefiting Vital Energy	(184)
Decoction of Arctii for Soothing Muscles	(186)
Decoction of Coptidis for Detoxification	(188)
Decoction of Cinnamomi Adding Cinnamomi	(189)
Decoction for General Antiphlogistic	(191)
Decoction for Purging Liver-fire and Eliminating Dampness	(192)
Golden Lock Bolus for Keep Kidney Essence	(194)
Zaizao Powder	(195)
Powder for Antiphlogosis	(197)
Pill of Six Miraculous Drugs	(199)
Decoction of Phragmitis	(201)
Powder of Lonicerae and Forsythiae	(202)
Powder of Ledebouriellae for Dispersing the Superficies	(204)
White Tiger Decoction	(206)
Decoction of Gypsum Fibrosum and Three Yellows	(207)
Decoction of Ginseng for Nourishing Qi and Ying	(208)
Ease Powder	(210)
Decoction of Aneglicae Pubescentis and Taxilli	(212)
Decoction for Pus Drainage and Relieving Pain	(214)
Xiaojin Pellet	(215)
Decoction for Warming Yang	(216)
Decoction of Persicae for Purgation	(218)
Major Decoction for Purging Down Digestive Qi	(219)
Major Decoction of Bupleurum	(221)
Pill of Stephaniae Tetrandrae, Zanthoxyli, Lepidii seu Descurainiae and Rhei	(222)
Powder of Bupleuri for Dispersing the Depressed Liver-Qi	(223)
Decoction of Gentianae for Purging Liver-Fire	(224)
Pulse-Activating Powder	(225)
Decoction for Rashes Subsidence	(226)
Decoction of Restoration	(228)
Decoction for Severe Phlegm-Heat Syndrome in the Chest	(229)
Decoction for Soothing the Intestine	(229)
Decoction of Angelicae Sinensis for Analgesic	(231)
Decoction of Angelicae Sinensis for Warming Cold Limbs	(232)
Decoction of Indigo Naturalis for Rashes Subsidence	(233)
Decoction of Sargassum for Goiter	(235)
Pill for Eliminating Phlegm Evil	(236)

Part One Treatment for Diseases

Chapter One
Ephelis

Ephelis, or freckle, is one of the small brownish spots in the skin that are usually due to precipitation of pigment and that increase in number and intensity on exposure to sunlight. In traditional Chinese medicine, it is due to insufficiency of kidney-essence resulting in ascending of asthenic fire along the meridians and stagnating on the face. Bad temper or intensive emotion may also change into *fire*-evil which may stagnate in collaterals due to attack of wind-evil. The main principle of the treatment is to invigorate kidney-yin to clear away fire-evil, disperse wind-evil and promote *blood* circulation. Ephelides may decrease in winter and increase in spring and summer. Preventing from sunlight and prohibition to peppery food is needed.

External Treatment

Recipe: *Yurong san*
Semen Phaseoli Radiati	300 g
Flos Nelumbinis	60 g
Talci	15 g
Radix Angelicae Dahuricae	15 g
Rhizoma Typhonii	15 g
Borneoli Synthetici	6 g
litharge	6 g

Grind the above drugs into fine powder. Apply it on the affected part after cleaning the face.

It is also effective for acne vulgaris and acne rosacea.

Ephelis

Recipe: *Mianshang hezi fang*
   Lignum Santali Albi

Grind *Lignum Santali Albi* to get juice. Apply the juice on the affected part.

Recipe: *Queban fang*
   jasmine seed

Dry the shelled seeds and grind them into powder. Mix it with a right amount of honey. Apply the mixture on the affected part.

Recipe: *Yangzhi queban liyu fang*
   Semen Pharbitidis
   egg white

Grind the seeds into powder and mix it with egg white. Apply the mixture on the affected part at bedtime, clean the face up the next morning. Keep away from eyebrows and lips.

Recipe: *Meirong gao*

Radix Ledebouriellae	60 g
Lignum Santali Albi	60 g
Rhizoma Ligustici	60 g
Rhizoma Bletillae	15 g
Rhizoma Typhonii	15 g
Radix Trichosanthis	15 g
Semen Phaseoli Radiati	15 g
Rhizoma Nardostachyos	15 g
Fructus Gleditsiae	a right amount
Lophanthus Rugosus	15 g

Grind the above drugs into fine powder and mix it with a right amount of honey. Apply the mixture on the face at bedtime. Suitable for oleaginous skin.

Recipe: *Yusanhua ye*
   Flos Lillii

Grind the flowers to get juice and rub the face with the juice, once daily.

Recipe: *Sigua san*

    towel gourd   60 g

Grind towel gourd into powder and apply it on the affected part.

Internal Treatment

Recipe: *Xijiao shengma wan*

Cornu Rhinocerotis	45 g
Rhizoma Cimicifugae	30 g
Rhizoma seu Radix Notopterygii	30 g
Radix Ledebouriellae	30 g
Rhizoma Typhonii	15 g
Radix Angelicae Dahuricae	15 g
Radix Rehmanniae	30 g
Rhizoma Ligustici Chuanxiong	15 g
Flos Carthami	15 g
Radix Scutellariae	15 g
Radix Glycyrrhizae	8 g

Grind the above drugs into fine powder. Steam it for one hour and make it into honeyed pills. Each weighs about 3 g. Take one pill with tea at bedtime, once daily.

30 cases with ephelides recovered completely after taking 6 to 18 doses. In the prescription, *Rhizoma seu Radix Notopterygii*, *Radix Ledebouriellae*, *Radix Angelicae Dahuricae*, *Rhizoma Cimicifugae*, *Rhizoma Typhonii* and *Radix Scutellariae* disperse wind-evil and clear away heat; *Cornu Rhinocerotis*, *Flos Carthami*, *Rhizoma Ligustici Chuanxiong* and *Radix Rehmanniae* cool *blood*-heat and remove blood stasis.

Recipe: *Liuwei dihuang wan*

Radix Rehmanniae Praeparata	24 g
Fructus Corni	12 g
Rhizoma Dioscoreae	12 g
Rhizoma Alismatis	12 g
Cortex Moutan Radicis	9 g

Ephelis

Poria   9 g

Grind the above drugs into fine powder and make it into honeyed pills. Each weighs about 3 g. Take 3 pills with warm water on an empty stomach. The dosage may be increased according to the constitution of the patient.

Chapter Two
Moth-Patch

Moth-patch is commonly seen in female cases, often occur during adolescent period, pregnancy or after pregancy. Also seen in cases with chronic hepatic disease, tuberculosis, tumor, irregular menstruation. According to traditional Chinese medicine, it is due to stagnation of liver-*qi* and blood stasis in the collaterals of the face resulting from depression; or insufficiency of *blood* resulting from deficiency of spleen-*qi*; or insufficiency of kidney-essence and asthenic heat stagnation resulting in incoordination between *qi* and *blood* on the face.

External Treatment

Recipe: *Wubai gao*

Rhizoma Bletillae	6 g
Radix Angelicae Dahuricae,	6 g
Radix Ampelopsis	4.5 g
Rhizoma Typhonii	6 g
Flos Caryophylli	4.5 g
lithrage	3 g

Grind the above drugs into fine powder and mix it with a right amount of egg white. Apply the mixture on the affected part at bedtime. Keep away from sunlight.

Recipe: *Bailian gao*

Radix Ampelopsis	15 g
lapis rubrum	15 g
Semen Armeniacae Amarum	15 g

Grind the above drugs into fine powder and mix it with a right amount of egg white. Apply the mixture on the affected part at bedtime. Keep away from sunlight.

Internal Treatment

Recipe: *Tusi quban tang*

Semen Cuscutae	15 g
Fructus Ligustri Lucidi	12 g
Herba Ecliptae	10 g
Radix Polygoni Multiflori	12 g
Radix Rehmanniae	15 g
Radix Rehmanniae Praeparata	15 g
Radix Paeoniae Alba	10 g
Radix Angelicae Sinensis	10 g
Colla Corii Asini	9 g
Fructus Lycii	9 g

All the above drugs are to be decocted in water for oral administration. One dose daily.

Recipe: *Xiao ban tang*

Radix Astragali seu Hedysari	15 – 18 g
Radix Codonopsis Pilosulae	9 – 12 g
Radix Angelicae Sinensis	9 – 15 g
Radix Paeoniae Rubra	9 – 15 g
Rhizoma Atractylodis Macrocephalae	9 – 12 g
Poria	9 – 12 g
Rhizoma Ligustici Chuanxiong	9 – 12 g
Radix Rehmanniae	9 – 12 g
Semen Persicae	10 g
Flos Carthami	10 g
Fructus Ziziphi Jujubae	10 dates
Radix Glycyrrhizae	6 g

All the above drugs are to be decocted in water for oral administration.

Ten doses consisted of one course of treatment. Two continuous courses suggested.

Recipe: *Hua ban tang*
Concha Margaitifera Usta	20 g
Bombyx Batryticatus	9 g
Flos Chrysanthemi	9 g
Herba Artemisiae Scopariae	12 g
Spica Prunellae	12 g
Retinervus Luffae Fructus	9 g
Radix Paeoniae Rubra	9 g
Radix Paeoniae Alba	9 g
Poria	12 g
Radix Glycyrrhizae	3 g
Herba Senecionis Scandentis	12 g

All the above drugs are to be decocted in water for oral administration. One dose daily.

This prescription is most suitable for cases during climacteric period.

Chapter Three
Acne

Acne is a disorder of the skin caused by inflammation of the skin glands and hair follicles. The disease is commonly seen during adolescence, more male cases than females. It often affects the face, upper chest and back. In traditional Chinese medicine, it is usually due to stagnation of heat evil in lung meridian or stagnation of blood-heat in the collaterals of face. Acne can be recurrent in many cases.

External Treatment

Recipe: *Gairong wan*

Bulbus Fritillariae Thunbergii	15 g
Rhizoma Typhonii	15 g
Radix Ledebouriellae	15 g
Folii Chrysanthemi	15 g
Talcum	15 g
Fructus Gleditsiae	50 g

Grind the above drugs into fine powder and make it into pills. Each weighs about 10 g. Mix one pill with a right amount of water and apply it on the affected part for 30 minutes. Then clean the face up. Twice daily.

Recipe: *Fushui gao*

Herba Spirodelae	150 g

Grind it into powder and mix it with honey. Apply the mixture on the affected part at bedtime. Clean up the face the next morning.

Recipe: *Zhi mianhufenci fang*

Chapter Three

    Semen Cuscutae   a right amount

Grind it to get juice. Apply the juice on the affected part at bedtime. Clean up the face the next morning.

Recipe: *Cuochuang chaji*

Sulfur	5 g
Alum	10 g
Radix et Rhizoma Rhei	5 g
Rhizoma Coptidis	3 g
Cortex Phellodendri	3 g

Grind the above drugs into powder and mix it with a right amount of water for washing the affected part. Twice daily.

20 cases with acne recovered completely after 7 to 25 days.

Recipe: *Shancigu san*

    Bulbus Iphigeniae   a right amount

Grind it into powder and mix it with a right amount of water for applying on the affected part.

Recipe: *Diandao san*

    Radix et Rhizoma Rhei
    Sulfur

Grind equal quantity of the drugs into powder and mix it with a right amount of water for applying on the affected part.

Internal Treatment

Recipe: *Pipa qingfei yin*

Radix Ginseng	2 g
Folium Eriobotryae	6 g
Radix Glycyrrhizae	2 g
Rhizoma Coptidis	3 g
Cortex Mori Radicis	6 g
Cortex Phellodendri	3 g

Acne

All the above drugs are to be decocted in water for oral administration. One dose daily.

Recipe: *Cuchuang ping tang*

Flos Lonicerae	15 g
Herba Taraxaci	15 g
Rhizoma Polygoni Cuspidati	2 g
Fructus Crataegi	12 g
Fructus Aurantii	10 g
Radix et Rhizoma Rhei	10 g

All the above drugs are to be decocted in water for oral administration. One dose daily.

Recipe: *Huayu sanjie wan*

Radix Angelicae Sinensis	60 g
Radix Paeoniae Rubra	60 g
Semen Persicae	30 g
Flos Carthami	30 g
Thallus Laminariae seu Eckloniae	30 g
Sargassi	30 g
Rhizoma Sparganii	30 g
Rhizoma Zedoariae	60 g
Spica Prunellae	60 g
Pericarpium Citri Reticulatae	60 g
Rhizoma Pinelliae	60 g

Grind the above drugs into fine powder and make it into pills with a right amount of water. Each weighs about 1 g. Take 9 pills each time, once daily.

In the prescription, *Radix Angelicae Sinensis*, *Semen Persicae*, *Flos Carthami*, *Rhizoma Sparganii*, *Rhizoma Zedoariae* can promote the circulation of blood to remove blood-stasis; *Thallus Laminariae seu Eckloniae*, *Sargassum*, *Spica Prunellae*, *Pericarpium Citri Reticulatae*, *Rhizoma Pinelliae* can dissolve phlegm stagnation. Contraindicated for cases during menstrual period or pregancy.

Recipe: Qing fei san

Fructus Forsythiae	2 g
Rhizoma Ligustici Chuanxiong	2 g
Radix Angelicae Dahuricae	2 g
Radix Scutellariae	2 g
Rhizoma Coptidis	2 g
Radix Glehniae	2 g
Herba Schizonepetae	2 g
Cortex Mori Radicis	2 g
Fructus Gardeniae	2 g
Bulbus Fritillariae Cirrhosae	2 g
Radix Glycyrrhizae	2 g

All the above drugs are to be decocted in water for oral administration. Take the decoction after meal, one dose daily.

In the prescription, *Radix Scutellariae*, *Rhizoma Coptidis*, *Fructus Gardeniae*, *Cortex Mori Radicis*, *Radix Glycyrrhizae* can clear away *fire* in the lung meridian; *Herba Schizonepetae* disperses wind-evil; *Bulbus Fritillariae Cirrhosae* dissolve the stagnation of phlegm; *Radix Glehniae* improves the production of bodily fluid.

Dietetic Treatment

Recipe: Pipa juhua zhou

Folium Eriobotryae	9 g
Flos Chrysanthemi	6 g
Gypsum Fibrosum	15 g
polished round – grained rice	60 g

Wrap the first three ingredients in a piece of gauze and decoct it in 300 ml of water until 200 ml of decoction is obtained. Add *polished round – grained rice* in the decoction and continue cooking until the gruel is done. Take the gruel once daily. It is effective for acne due to heat stagnation in the lung and stomach meridians.

Recipe: Taoren shanzha zhou

Acne

Semen Persicae	9 g
Fructus Crataegi	9 g
Bulbus Fritillariae Cirrhosae	9 g
Folium Nelumbinis	6 g
polished round – grained rice	60 g

Decoct the first four ingredients and filter the decoction when it is done. Add *polished round – grained rice* in the decoction and continue cooking until the gruel is done. Take the gruel once daily. It is most effective for acne tuberata.

Acupuncture

1. **Puncture Qūchí(LI11) and Hégǔ(LI4)** with moderate stimulation. Retain the needles for 30 minutes after needling sensation is obtained. Rotating and twisting method is applied 3 to 4 times during needle-retaining period. 10 continuous days of treatment consisted of one course.

2. Prickling and cupping therapy is applied to **DàZhuī(DU14)**. The cup is retained for 10 to 15 minutes. Once every 3 days.

Others

Recipe 1
Ingredients
   red sage root (*Radix Salviae Miltiorrhizae*)   100 g

Process   Grind it into fine powder, then store it in a bottle for later use.
Directions   Take it three times daily, 3 g for each time.

Recipe 2
Ingredients
   loquat leaf (*Folium Eriobotryae*)
   prunella spike (*Spica Prunellae*)
   mulberry bark (*Cortex Mori Radicis*)
   honeysuckle flower (*Flos Lonicerae*)
   forsythia fruit (*Fructus Forsythiae*)

      scutellaria root (*Radix Scutellariae*)
      bryozoatum
      liquorice (*Radix Glycyrrhizae*)

    Process Decoct all the ingredients twice in water, sift out the decoctions and mix them well.

    Directions Take it in twice, one dose daily.

Recipe 3

Ingredients

red sage root (*Radix Salviae Miltiorrhizae*)	15 g
scutellaria root (*Radix Scutellariae*)	12 g
raw capejasmine fruit (*Fructus Gardeniae*)	12 g
mulberry bark (*Cortex Mori Radicis*)	12 g
Moutan bark (*Cortex Moutan Radicis*)	12 g
red peony root (*Radix Paeoniae Rubra*)	12 g
forsythia fruit (*Fructus Forsythiae*)	9 g
rhubarb (*Radix et Rhizoma Rhei*)	3 g
raw liquorice (*Radix Glycyrrhizae*)	3 g

    Process Decoct them in right amount of water twice, sift out the decoctions and mix them well.

    Directions Take it in twice daily, one dose daily.

Recipe 4

Ingredients

raw hawthorn fruit (*Fructus Crataegi*)	30 g
reed Rhizome (*Rhizoma Phragmitis*)	30 g
crystal sugar	right amount

    Process Decoct them in right amount of water.

    Directions Take the decoction as drink, twice daily.

Treatment for Acne Rosacea

    Recipe: *Zhi bichi fang*
      Radix et Rhizoma Rhei

Acne

    Natrii Sulphas
    Semen Arecae

Grind the above drugs into fine powder and apply it on the affected part (mixed with a right amount of water), three to four times daily.

Recipe: *Bailian san*
    Radix Ampelopsis
    lapis rubrum
    Semen Armeniacae Amarum

Grind the above drugs into fine powder and apply it on the affected part (mixed with a right amount of egg white) at bedtime. Clean the nose the next morning.

Recipe: *Zhizi wan*

Fructus Gardeniae	200 g
Rhizoma Ligustici Chuanxiong	120 g
Radix et Rhizoma Rhei	180 g
Semen Sojae Praeparatum	200 g
Radix Glycyrrhizae	120 g

Grind the above drugs into fine powder and make it into honeyed pills. Each weighs about 1 g. Take 10 to 15 pills each time, three times daily. It is effective for acne rosacea due to blood-stasis in combination with heat evil stagnating in the nose. Contraindicated for cases with deficiency of the spleen and stomach.

Recipe: *Lingxiaohua san*
    Flos Campsis Grandiflora
    Fructus Gardeniae

Grind equal amount of the above drugs into fine powder and take 6 g with tea after meals. It is effective for acne rosacea due to sthenic heat evil stagnating in the *blood*. Contraindicated for cases with deficiency of the spleen and stomach. Pregnant women prohibited.

Recipe: *Liangxue siwu tang*

Radix Angelicae Sinensis	3 g
Radix Rehmanniae	3 g
Rhizoma Ligustici Chuanxiong	3 g
Radix Paeoniae Rubra	3 g
Radix Scutellariae	3 g
Poria	3 g
Pericarpium Citri Reticulatae	3 g
Flos Carthami	3 g
Radix Glycyrrhizae	3 g
Faeces Trogopterori	6 g

Decoct the first nine drugs in 300 ml of water until 200 ml of decoction obtained. Take the decoction with powder of *Faeces Trogopterori* and a right amount of millet wine. 6 g of *Radix Astragali seu Hedysari* required in case of *qi*-deficiency seen. It is suitable for acne rosacea due to heat evil and blood-stasis in the nose.

Recipe: *Dongguazi san*

Semen Benincase	30 g
Semen Biotae	30 g
Poria	30 g
Radix Semiaquilegiae	30 g
Fructus Aurantii Immaturus	30 g
Fructus Gardeniae	60 g

Grind the above drugs into fine powder and take 6 g after meals. Effective for acne rosacea at the initial stage and middle stage.

Recipe: *Chilong san*

Lapis Rubri	75 g
Radix Ledebouriellae	60 g
Radix Paeoniae Rubra	60 g
Cortex Lycii Radicis	60 g
Radix Polygoni Multiflori	60 g
Radix Angelicae Sinensis	60 g
Fructus Gardeniae	60 g

Acne

Radix Glycyrrhizae   30 g

Grind the above drugs into fine powder and take 6 g with warm millet wine after meals. Effective for acne rosacea due to wind-heat evil stagnating in the lung meridian.

Chapter Four
Wart

Wart Warts are the benign skin vegetations caused by virus infection and autoinoculation. In this group of skin diseases, there are the common warts, plantar warts, flat warts, infectious soft warts and pointed condyloma. All of them can be treated by foot acupuncture, except pointed condyloma.

According to traditional Chinese medicinehe, liver can store blood and control tendons; and the spleen is in charge of digestion and it can control limbs and muscles. In patients with deficiency of liver and with dryness in blood, the tendons and blood vessels can not obtain enough nutrition; the invaded external wind and heat pathogens may be retained in skin and muscle to cause stagnation of qi and blood to produce the warts. The spleen is in charge of digestion and it can control limbs. In patients with deficiency of spleen, the excessive dampness pathogen may be accumulated to block circulation of qi to produce the warts.

External Treatment

Recipe: *Shenmian youzi fang*
Rhizoma Arisaematis   a right amount

Grind the above drugs into fine powder and mix it with a right amount of edible vinegar. Apply the mixture on the affected part.

Recipe: *Xiao you gao*
Retinervus Luffae Fructus   10 g
edible salt   a right amount

Mix the ingredients and pound it into mash. Apply it on the affected part and rub the warts until the skin is congested.

Wart

Recipe: *Youxi fang*

Herba Portulacae	60 g
Nidus Vespae	9 g
Radix Angelicae Dahuricae	9 g
Fructus Cnidii	9 g
Herba Asari	9 g
Pericarpium Citri Reticulatae	15 g
Rhizoma Atractylodis	15 g
Radix Sophorae Flavescentis	15 g

Decoct the ingredients and filter the decoction when it is done. Wash the warts with the warm decoction for 15 minutes, four to five times daily.

In the prescription, *Herba Portulacae* can clear away heat-evil and resolve swelling; *Nidus Vespae* can remove toxic evil; *Radix Angelicae Dahuricae*, *Fructus Cnidii*, *Herba Asari*, *Radix Sophorae Flavescentis* can disperse wind-evil and clear away heat; *Pericarpium Citri Reticulatae* and *Rhizoma Atractylodis* can dissolve dampness.

Internal Treatment

Recipe: *Quyou fang*

Herba Portulacae	60 g
Herba Patriniae	15 g
Radix Arnebiae seu Lithospermi	15 g
Folium Isatidis	15 g

All the above drugs are to be decocted in water for oral administration. One dose daily. Seven days of treatment consisted of one course.

In the prescription, *Herba Portulacae* is effective for clearing away heat-evil. *Herba Patriniae* and *Folium Isatidis* can help clear away heat-toxin. *Radix Arnebiae seu Lithospermi* can cool blood-heat.

Recipe: *Honghua quyou tang*

Flos Carthami	10 g

Soak the drug in boiling water and drink it instead of tea when it is warm.

Three times daily. 10 days of treatment consisted of one course.

 Recipe: *Daqing yiyiren tang*

Haematitum	30 g
Os Draconis	30 g
Concha Ostreae	30 g
Semen Coicis	30 g
Herba Portulacae	30 g
Folium Isatidis	12 g
Radix Angelicae Sinensis	12 g
Radix Paeoniae Rubra	12 g
Radix Salviae Miltiorrhizae	12 g
Rhizoma Cimicifugae	6 g

All the above drugs are to be decocted in water for oral administration. One dose daily.

Folium Isatidis, *Herba Portulacae* and *Semen Coicis* are commonly used to treat warts. *Radix Angelicae Sinensis* along with *Radix Salviae Miltiorrhizae* and *Radix Paeoniae Rubra* promote blood circulation and remove blood stasis. *Haematitum*, *Os Draconis* and *Concha Ostreae* can calm liver-yang and restrain the ascending of liver-*fire*. *Rhizoma Cimicifugae* can clear away heat-toxin and disperse supeficial evil.

Dietetic Treatment

 Recipe: *Yimi baihe zhou*

Semen Coicis	30 g
Bulbus Lillii	6 g

Cook the ingredients in a right amount of water over fire to make gruel. Take the gruel prior to breakfast and supper, twice daily.

Acupuncture

Puncture **Dàgǔkōng(EX – UE5)** and retain the needles for 30 minutes after needling sensation is got. Electro-acupuncture can be applied during needle-retaining stage. Once daily. One course consists of 5 days of treatment. There is an interval of 3 to 4 days between two courses.

Chapter Five
Peripheral Facial Paralysis

Peripheral facial paralysis, or Bell's palsy is a paralysis of one side of the face, is facial paralysis which occurs suddenly and mostly after exposure to cold wind or trauma. It may occur at any age but is slightly more common in the age group from 20 to 50. 85 – 90% of the patients get recovered spontaneously. In traditional Chinese medicine, the onset of the illness is thought to be due to derangement of qi and blood and malnutrition of the channels caused by invasion of the channels and collaterals in the facial region by pathogenic wind – cold or phlegm. If falls into the category of "zhen zhong feng", "kou yan wai xie" or "diao xian feng" (deviation of the eye and mouth) in traditional Chinese medicine.

Etiology and Pathogenesis

The paralysis of facial muscles is caused by the attack of wind cold or wind heat pathogen to the meridians of face and the stagnation of qi in meridians or due to the invasion of damp – heat pathogen from liver and gallbladder to the meridians.

Main Points of Diagnosis

1. It often occurs in autumn and winter or between spring and summer, mostly in the middle – aged. The disease usually attacks one side of the face.
2. The diagnosis is based on the symptoms, but most rule out cerebrovascular accidents (strokes) and intracranial tumors. The peripheral facial paralysis patients are specially unable to frown and raise the eyebrow, close the eye of

the paralyzed side. The intracranial tumors can be ruled out X – ray examination.

3. The attack comes all of a sudden. At the beginning the patient feels numb at one side of the face, pain around the ear and tenderness in the mastoidal region. Then the mouth becomes wry, the nasolabial groove no longer seen and the facio-buccal region relaxed and strengthless. It is impossible to have the cheeks blown up. The eyeballs are still exposed when the eyes are shut. It is difficult to frown and speak. Salivation comes down from the corners of the mouth. The sense of taste is lost but the sense of hearing is hypersensitive. There may be pain in the mastoid region or headache.

Differential Diagnosis and Treatment

1) Wind heat pathogen

The patients may suffer from headache, deviation of mouth and eye, lacrimation, dripping of saliva, fever, chillness, burning pain and redness in ear root, annoyance, dryness and bitter taste in mouth, dark urine and constipation. The tongue proper is red in color with yellow and greasy coating and the pulse is floating and rapid.

Therapeutic principle   To expel wind, clear heat and release stasis in collaterals.

Principal acupoints   **Hégǔ(LI4)** and **Qiántóudiǎn**.

Supplemental acupoints   **Shāngyáng(LI1), Láogōng(PC8)**.

2) Wind cold pathogen

The patients may suffer from deviation of mouth and eye, hatred of coldness to face, pale complexion, severe pain in the ear root, headache, poor appetite and long stream of clear urine. The tongue proper is pale with thin and white coating and the pulse is floating and tense.

Therapeutic principle   To expel wind and cold pathogen and release stasis in the collaterals.

Principal acupoints   **Yángchí(SJ4), Shàofǔ(HT8)**.

Supplemental acupoints   **Nèiguān(PC6), Wàiguān(SJ5)**.

Body Acupuncture Therapy

Points   Yìfēng(SJ17), Dìcāng(ST4), Jiáchē(ST6), Yángbái(GB14), Tàiyáng(EX-HN5), Hégǔ(LI4), Quánliáo(SI18) and Xiàguān(ST7).

Method   3 to 5 of the above points are selected for each treatment and the therapy is given once daily. Dìcāng(ST4) and Jiáchē(ST6) are punctured together with one needle inserted horizontally from Dìcāng(ST4) to Jiáchē(ST6). The following points can also be added to the formula according to the symptoms: Fēngchí(GB20) for headache; Fēnglóng(ST40) for profuse sputum; Cuánzhú(BL2) and Sīzhúkōng(SJ23) for difficulty in frowning and raising the eyebrow; Cuánzhú(BL2), Jīngmíng(BL1), Tóngzǐliáo(GB1), Yúyāo(EX-HN4) and Sīzhúkōng(SJ23) for incomplete closing of the eyelids; Yíngxiāng(LI20) for difficulty in sniffing; Shuǐgōu(DU26) for deviation of the philtrum; Jūliáo(GB29) for inability to show the teeth; Tīnghuì(GB2) for tinnitus and deafness; Wàngǔ(SI4) for tenderness at the mastoid region; and Tàichōng(LR3) for twitching of the eyelid and the mouth.

Electro-acupuncture Therapy

Main Points   Qianzheng(an extra-point) and Yìfēng(SJ17).

Auxiliary Points   Yángbái(GB14), Tàiyáng(EX-HN5) and Dìcāng(ST4).

Method   One of the main points and two or three of the auxiliary points are prescribed each time. The main point is connected to the negative pole of the electro-acupuncture machine, and the auxiliary points to the positive pole. The frequency is adjusted to 20 to 30 times per minute with an output which can just cause the muscular twitch on the affected side. The treatment lasts for 15 minutes and is repeated once every other day. Ten times consisted of one course.

The patient can be assured that recovery usually occurs in 2 to 8 weeks (or up to one to two years in older patients). In the vast majority of cases, partial or complete recovery occurs. When recovery is partial, contractures may develop on the paralyzed side. Recurrence on the same or the opposite side is occasionally reported.

Other External Treatment

1) Apply adhesive plaster on the acupoints   Dust 0.5 to 1 gram of the powder of Semen Strychni onto a plaster and then apply the plaster on the acupoint of Tàiyáng(EX-HN5), Xiàguān(ST7) and Jiáchē(ST6) of the affected side

(more applicable to the regions with tenderness). Change the plaster every 3 days. If blisters appear on the administered part, extract its fluid after disinfection. Then the blisters will get cured spontaneously.

2) Smear the blood of eel onto the affected region Smear fresh blood of eel onto the buccal skin of the affected side, and hold the mouth angle of the affected side with a metal hook so as to help cure the facial paralysis. This is to be done once a day.

3) Do local massage on the affected region, several times a day.

Therapeutic Methods by Practising Qigong
1. Self - Treatment by Practising Qigong
1) Basic Maneuvers
It is advisable to practise Head and Face Qigong.
2) Auxiliary Maneuvers
Those shedding tears ought to lay emphasis on kneading **Yángbái(GB14)**, **Sìbái(ST2)**, and **Tóngzǐliáo(GB1)**.

At the initial stage, the pressing and kneading manipulations applied locally should be light; as for those with a long course of disease, the manipulations should be heavier.

2. External Qi Therapy
1) Basic Maneuvers
(1) Press and knead the acupoints **Yángbái (GB14)**, **Chéngqì (ST1)**, **Sīzhúkōng (SJ23)**, **Tóngzǐliáo (GB1)**, **Tīnggōng (SI19)**, **Yìfēng (SJ17)**, **Quánliáo (SI18)**, **Yíngxiāng(LI20)**, **Jiáchē(ST6)**, **Fēngchí(GB20)** and **Hégǔ(LI4)**.

(2) Apply the flat - palm form, use the pushing, pulling and leading manipulations to emit qi onto the unilateral paralyzed face, conduct the channel qi from front to back and along the Large Intestine Meridian to the terminals of the upper extremities.

2) Auxiliary Maneuvers
In the anaphase of the paralysis, the additional application of the vibrating and quivering manipulation is advised to provoke the channel qi.

Treatment by Chinese Massage
There will be gradual recovery in on or two weeks after its onset. Manipulation of massage may help the recovery of facial nerves and muscular function

and reduce sequelae. During the treatment, stimulus of cold to the face and head should be avoided and the patient should knead the face frequently for enhancing the effectiveness.

1. Manipulation   Pushing with one-finger meditation, digital-pressing, pressing, grasping and kneading.

2. Location of Points: **Hégǔ**(LI4), **Qūchí**(LI11), **Xiàguān**(ST7), **Jiáchē**(ST6), **Yìfēng**(SJ17), **Tàiyáng**(EX-HN5), **Jīngmíng**(BL1), **Sìbái**(ST2), **Yíngxiāng**(LI20), **Shuǐgōu**(DU26) and **Dìcāng**(ST4).

3. Operation

1) The doctor stands in front and to the side of the sitting patient and holds the posterolateral part of the head with one hand. Using one-finger meditation pushing or thumb-pressing-kneading, the doctor pushes with the other hand repeatedly from **Yìntáng**(EX-HN3) along the supercilliary of the affected side to **Tàiyáng**(EX-HN5) for 2 or 3 times first; then pushes repeatedly from **Yìntáng**(EX-HN3) upwards by way of **Shéntíng**(DU24) to **Bǎihuì**(DU20) also for 2 or 3 times; finally, pushes repeatedly from the middle of the forehead via **Yángbái**(GB14) of the affected part to **Tàiyáng**(EX-HN5) for 2 or 3 times.

2) After that, in the above-mentioned way, the doctor pushes downwards repeatedly from Yintang(EX-HN3) by way of **Jīngmíng**(BL1) of the affected side, along the side of the nose up to **Yingxiang**(LI20) for 2 or 3 times. Then the doctor pushes from **Yíngxiāng**(LI20), along the point of **Sìbái**(ST2), **Quánliáo**(SI18), **Xiàguān**(ST7) and **Jiáchē**(ST6) passing the face, to **Dìcāng**(ST4) at the labial angle.

3) Still in the same way mentioned above, the operator pushes from **Dìcāng**(ST4) to **Shuǐgōu**(DU26) circling the lips, by way of **Chéngjiāng**(RN24), and returns to the starting point. Then the operator pushes along the mandible to **Jiáchē**(ST6). Finally rub and scrub softly the affected side of the face with the palm till local warmth and heat are produced.

In the above-mentioned operations, the movement of the hand should pass at every point with a bit more strength exerted and some stimulating manipulations such as digit-pressing used in combination.

4) The doctor stands to the side of the patient and, with one hand holding his forehead, grasps **Fēngchí**(GB20) and the tendons of the back nape up and down repeatedly for three to five times, finally pushes the point Qiaogong for

30 times.

5) The doctor standing behind the patient, grasps **Jiānjǐng(GB21)** with two hands and in an orderly way presses and kneads **Qūchí(LI11)** and **Hégǔ (LI4)**.

4. Course of Treatment   Once a day, six days for one course with an interval of 3 days between two courses.

Chapter Six
Thyroid Adenoma

Thyroid adenoma is a common benign tumor of the neck. It belongs to the category of *rou ying* (fleshy tumor) in traditional Chinese medicine. It usually occurs in people from 20 to 40 years old and is most common in female.

Main Points of Diagnosis

1. There is an individual lump in the front part of the neck. It is soft, smooth and well limited. When the patient swallows, it moves up and down.
2. There are not any symptoms present. The lump itself grows very slowly. In most cases it does not get larger for many years. If it happens to bleed in a cystadenoma, the lump will increase very quickly accompanied with distending pain, pressing sensation and uncomfortable feeling.
3. A large thyroid adenoma may compress the trachea and causes distress and disturbance in respiration.
4. **Isotopic Iodine**[131] Scanning shows that the adenoma is mostly a warm nodule while the cyst is mostly a cool nodule. On ultrasonography reflection of liquid segment will be seen. If the liquid in the cyst is thick and sticky, tiny wave may be found in liquid segment.

Differentiation and Treatment of Common Syndromes

1. **External Treatment**
1) **application**
Apply *Yanghe jiening gao* (*Paste for activating yang and resolving coagulation of yin*) mixed with *Heitui paste for treating all abscesses of yin syndromes*) onto the affected part.
Recipe: *Yanghe jiening gao*

Thyroid Adenoma

Fructus et Radix et Folium et Caulis Arctii	1500 g
Caulis Impatientis	124 g
Rhizoma Chuanxiong	124 g
Radix Aconiti Lateralis Praeparata	60 g
Caulis Cinnamomi	60 g
Radix et Rhizoma Rhei	60 g
Cortex Cinnamomi	60 g
Radix Aconiti Kusnezoffi	60 g
Lumbricus	60 g
Bombyx Batryticatus	60 g
Radix Paeoniae Rubra	60 g
Radix Angelicae Dahuricae	60 g
Radix Ampelopsis	60 g
Rhizoma Bletillae	60 g
Olibanum	60 g
Myrrha	60 g
Radix Dipsaci	30 g
Saposhinkoviae	30 g
Herba Schizonepetae	30 g
Faeces Trogopterori	30 g
Radix Aucklandiae	30 g
Pericarpium Citri	30 g
Pericarpium Citri Reticulatae	30 g
storax oil	120 g
Moschus	30 g
Oleum Sesami	5000 g

2) **acupuncture**

The acupuncture point is Dingchuan(**EX - B1**). Apply the treatment once every two days.

3) **operative treatment**

After having been treated with traditional Chinese drugs for three months, if the lump is not reduced obviously or is associated with severe hyperthyroidism or has obvious compressing symptoms or is very hard, an operation should be carried out.

2. Internal Treatment

1) the type of stagnancy of phlegm and qi

Main Symptoms and Signs: There is an individual lump in the front part of the neck, hemispheric in shape and smooth on the surface. When touched upon, the lump is painless and can move up and down as the patient swallows, associated with distress and distention in the chest and stuffiness in the throat, thin and greasy fur on the tongue and taut and rapid pulse.

Therapeutic Principles: Regulating the flow of qi to alleviate mental depression and removing phlegm to resolve masses.

Recipe: *Haizao yuhu tang* (*Decoction of Sargassum for resolving masses*)

Sargassum	15 g
Thallus Eckloniae	15 g
Bulbus Fritillariae Thunbergii	10 g
Fructus Forsythiae	10 g
Rhizoma Pinelliae Praeparata	10 g
Pericarpium Citri Reticulatae Viride	10 g
Radix Angelicae Pubescentis	10 g
Rhizoma Ligustici Chuanxiong	10 g
Radix Angelica Sinensis	10 g
Radix Glycyrrhizae	10 g

Decoct the above ingredients in a right amount of water for oral administration.

For those who suffer from distress and disorder in the chest, add 10 grams of *Rhizoma Cyperi* and *Radix Curcumae Kwangsiensis* each. For those with hard masses, add 10 grams of *Spica Prunellae*, *Rhizoma Pleionis* each and 10 grams of *Rhizoma Dioscoreae Bulbiferae*.

2) the type of deficiency of the spleen and stagnation of the liver-qi

Main Symptoms and Signs: There are nodules in the local affected area, accompanied with mental depression, fullness and discomfort in the chest, irritability and impetuosity, abdominal distention and loss of appetite, loose stool and edema, pale tongue with thin whitish fur and taut and thready pulse.

Therapeutic Principles: Soothing the liver, invigorating the spleen, and removing phlegm to resolve masses.

Recipe: *Xiaoyao san* (*Ease powder*)

Radix Bupleuri	15 g
Radix Angelicae Sinensis	15 g
Radix Paeoniae Alba	15 g
Poria	15 g
Rhizoma Atractylodis Macrocephalae	15 g
Radix Glycyrrhizae	10 g
Rhizoma Zingiberis Recens	3 pcs
Herba Menthae	6 g

Decoct the above ingredients in a right amount of water for oral administration.

For removing phlegm to resolve masses, add 10 grams of *Pericarpium Citri Reticulatae* and *Rhizoma Pinelliae Praeparata* each, 15 grams of *Sargassum*, *Thallus Eckloniae* each and 15 grams of *Spica Prunellae*.

3) **fire-toxin type**

Main Symptoms and Signs: It is seen in those who have adenoma complicated with cystous bleeding and infection. The manifestations are fever, speedy enlargement of the lump, redness, swelling, heat and pain in the local affected part, reddish tongue with yellow fur, slippery and rapid pulse.

Therapeutic Principles: Clearing away pathogenic heat and toxic materials, cooling the blood to stop bleeding.

Recipe: Qingye zicao tang (Decoction of Isatis leaf and Arnebia)

Folium Isatidis	15 g
Herba Taraxaci	15 g
Herba Agrimoniae	15 g
Fructus Forsythiae	15 g
Rhizoma Coptidis	10 g
Cortex Moutan Radicis	10 g
Spica Prunellae	10 g
Radix Arnebiae seu Lithospermi	10 g
Radix et Rhizoma Rhei	10 g

Decoct the above ingredients in a right amount of water for oral administration.

Chapter Seven
Calvities

Calvities, or baldness, refers to the state of being lacking all or significant part of the hair on the head or sometimes on other parts of the body. It is divided into two types in traditional Chinese medicine: sthenic and deficient types. The former is usually caused by the attack of wind, cold, dampness, dryness, phlegm, stasis or other evils being stagnant in the hair roots leading to difficulty of *qi* and *blood* circulation resulting in malnutrition of the hair. The latter is due to deficiency of liver-*yin* and kidney-*yin* or insufficiency of *yin-blood* leading to malnutrition of hair.

The treatment should prevent the baldness and promote regeneration of hair in the mead time.

External Treatment

Recipe: *Xifa juhua san*

Flos Chrysanthemi	30 g
Fructus Viticis	30 g
Cacumen Biotae	30 g
Rhizoma Ligustici Chuanxiong	30 g
Cortex Mori Radicis	30 g
Radix Angelicae Dahuricae	30 g
Herba Asari	30 g
Herba Ecliptae	30 g

All the above drugs are decocted in water. Wash the hair and the bald part with the decoction.

It is effective for baldness due to the attack of wind-evil in the hair roots. *Flos Chrysanthemi*, *Rhizoma Ligustici Chuanxiong*, *Fructus Viticis*, *Radix Angelicae Dahuricae*, *Herba Asari*, *Cacumen Biotae* can disperse wind-evil on the head and face. *Herba Ecliptae* and *Cortex Mori Radicis* can promote the regeneration of hair.

Recipe: Hai'ai tang

Folium Artemisiae Argyi	6 g
Flos Chrysanthemi	6 g
Herba Menthae	6 g
Radix Ledebouriellae	6 g
Rhizoma Ligustici	6 g
Rhizoma Nardostachyos	6 g
Lophanthus Rugosus	6 g
Fructus Viticis	6 g
Herba Schizonepetae	6 g

Decoct the above ingredients in a right amount of water. Wash hair with the decoction.

This prescription is effective for alopecia areata due to the attack of wind-heat in combination with *blood*-deficiency.

Recipe: Shengfa wuyun you

Radix Gentianae Macrophyllae	30 g
Radix Angelicae Dahuricae	30 g
Rhizoma Ligustici Chuanxiong	30 g
Fructus Viticis	15 g
Lignum Santali Albi	15 g
Radix Aconiti Praeparata	15 g

Pound the drugs into crude powder, wrap it in a piece of gauze and soak it in a right amount of sesame oil for 21 days. Apply the medicated oil on the affected part, three times daily. Rub the scalp until the skin is congested.

This prescription is effective for alopecia due to stagnation of wind, cold and dampness-evil in hair roots resulting in malnutrition of hair. *Radix Gentianae Macrophyllae* and *Radix Aconiti Praeparata* can disperse wind-cold in meridians and collaterals; *Radix Angelicae Dahuricae*, *Rhizoma Ligustici Chuanxiong*, *Fructus Viticis* can disperse wind evil in the head; *Lignum Santali Albi* promotes qi circulation in the collaterals.

Recipe: *Zhitu shengfa fang*
  Semen Cannabis   a right amount
  Radix Gentianae Macrophyllae   a right amount

Decoct the drugs in a right amount of water. Wash hair with the decoction.

Recipe: *Zhangfa zirong san*
  Rhizoma Zingiberis Recens   30 g
  Radix Ginseng   30 g

Cut *Rhizoma Zingiberis Recens* into slices and grind *Radix Ginseng* into powder. Rub the affected part with slices of ginger and powder of ginseng.

Recipe: *Shuanghua erwu ding*
  Flos Genkwa   3 g
  Flos Carthami   3 g
  Radix Aconiti   6 g
  Herba Asari   3 g
  Pericarpium Zanthoxyli   3 g

Grind the above drugs into fine powder and soak it in 75% alcohol in a sealed bottle for one week. Apply the tincture on the bald part and rub the skin until it is congested. Once daily. One course of treatment consists of thirty days.

This prescription is effective for alopecia areata due to stagnation of cold-dampness in hair roots. It can help promote qi and blood circulation and remove blood-stasis.

Internal Treatment

Recipe: *Shenying yangzhen dan*
  Rhizoma seu Radix Notopterygii

Calvities

    Cydonia Lagenaria
    Rhizoma Gastrodiae
    Radix Paeoniae Alba
    Radix Angelicae Sinensis
    Semen Cuscutae
    Rhizoma Ligustici Chuanxiong
    Radix Rehmanniae Praeparata

    Grind the above drugs into fine powder and make it into honeyed pills. Each weighs about 1 g. Take 30 pills with salt wate on an empty stomach.

    In this prescription, **Radix Angelicae Sinensis**, **Radix Rehmanniae Praeparata**, **Radix Paeoniae Alba**, **Rhizoma Ligustici Chuanxiong** can promote the production and circulation of *blood*, also effective for invigorating liver and kidney combining with **Semen Cuscutae**. **Rhizoma Gastrodiae**, **Rhizoma seu Radix Notopterygii**, **Cydonia Lagenaria** can disperse the attack of wind evil and calm hyperactivity of liver-*yang*. The prescription is suitable for cases with calvities due to wind-dryness and *blood*-deficiency.

    Recipe: Zhi bantu fang

Radix Rehmanniae	15 g
Radix Rehmanniae Praeparata	15 g
Caulis Spatholobi	15 g
Herba Polygoni Multiflori	15 g
Radix Paeoniae Alba	15 g
Fructus Mori	15 g
Radix Astragali seu Hedysari	30 g
Rhizoma Ligustici Chuanxiong	9 g
Herba Ecliptae	9 g
Rhizoma Gastrodiae	6 g
Cordyceps	6 g
Chinese flowering quince	6 g

    All the above drugs are decocted in water for oral administration. One dose daily. It is most effecive for alopecia of deficient type.

    Recipe: Tongqiao huoxue tang

Radix Paeoniae Rubra	3 g
Rhizoma Ligustici Chuanxiong	3 g
Semen Persicae	9 g
Flos Carthami	9 g
Bulbus Allii Fistulosi	9 g
Rhizoma Zingiberis Recens	9 g
Fructus Ziziphi Jujubae	7
Moschus	1.5 g

Decoct the first seven ingredients in 250 ml of millet wine until 200 ml of decoction obtained. Remove the dregs and add in moschus. Continue the decoction for two minutes.

This prescription is most effective for alopecia due to blood stasis in upper-jiao and blood-stasis in the head due to trauma(ta). *Flos Carthami*, *Semen Persicae*, *Radix Paeoniae Rubra*, *Rhizoma Ligustici Chuanxiong* promote blood circulation and remove *blood*-deficiency. *Fructus Ziziphi Jujubae*, *Rhizoma Zingiberis Recens* and *Bulbus Allii Fistulosi* disperse stagnation and promote qi and blood circulation in the collateral and superficies. *Moschus* leads other drugs to the diseased parts.

Recipe: *Erxian wan*

Cacumen Biotae	240 g
Radix Angelicae Sinensis	120 g

Grind the above drugs into fine powder and make it into honeyed pills. Each weighs about 1 g. Take 30 pills each time, twice daily. It is suitable for alopecia due to *blood*-heat resulting in malnutrition of hair.

Recipe: *Yangyin xiehuo tang*

Radix Rehmanniae	12 g
Cortex Moutan Radicis	6 g
Cortex Phellodendri	6 g
Radix Paeoniae Rubra	9 g
Poria	9 g
Rhizoma Dioscoreae	9 g
Fructus Corni	9 g

Rhizoma Anemarrhenae 9 g
Rhizoma Achyranthis Bidentatae 9 g
Rhizoma Ligustici Chuanxiong 3 g

All the above drugs are to be decocted in water for oral administration. One dose daily.

This prescription is effective for cases with alopecia deu to *yin*-deficiency of kidney causing hyperactivity of *yang*. The patient may manifest emaciation, epistaxis, soreness sensation of the waist and knees, restlessness, insomnia and emission; red tongue with little fur, thin, rapid pulse. The presentation of alopecia is similar to seborrheic alopecia.

Recipe: Fuling zhu san

Rhizoma Atractylodis Macrocephalae 480 g
Poria 120 g
Rhizoma Alismatis 120 g
Polyporus Umbellatus 120 g
Cortex Cinnamomi 240 g

Grind the above drugs into fine powder. Take 10 g each time, three times daily. It is effective for alopecia due to spleen deficiency leading to stagnation of dampness evil in hair roots.

Recipe: Qing fei sheng fa tang

Cortex Mori Radicis 9 g
Cortex Lycii Radicis 9 g
Radix Scutellariae 9 g
Semen Cannabis 9 g
Semen Biotae 9 g
Radix Polygoni Multiflori 9 g
Frucus Xanthii 9 g
Rhizoma Anemarrhenae 9 g
Radix Rehmanniae 9 g
Cortex Moutan Radicis 9 g
Rhizoma Imperatae 30 g
Radix Glycyrrhizae 15 g

All the above drugs are to be decocted in water for oral administration. One dose daily.

This prescription is effective for alopecia due to hyperactivity of lung-heat resulting in malnutrition of hair and skin. *Cortex Mori Radicis*, *Radix Scutellariae*, *Frucus Xanthii* clear away sthenic heat in the lung meridian; *Rhizoma Anemarrhenae* and *Cortex Lycii Radicis* clear away asthenic heat in the lung; *Semen Cannabis*, *Semen Biotae*, *Radix Polygoni Multiflori* and *Radix Rehmanniae* invigorate *yin* and moisturize dryness; *Cortex Moutan Radicis* and *Rhizoma Imperatae* clear away heat in the *blood* and promote blood circulation.

Acupuncture

Plum-blossom needle is used to tap the affected part after strict disinfection. Mild bleeding required.

Chapter Eight
Simple Obesity

Simple obesity is a common phenomenon in people of all ages. Simple obesity refers to non-pathologic adiposity. The body weight of such patients is 20% heavier than the body weight based on the criteria recommended by WHO.

The normal way of calculation of body-weight is:

Male standard body weight (kg) = (height of a person(cm) - 100) × 1
Female standard body weight (kg) = (height of a person(cm) - 100) × 0.9
Standard body weight of child (kg) = Age × 2 + 8
Another normal way of calculation is as follows:
Body - height (cm) - 100/105 = the standard body weight of man/woman.

Etiology and Pathogenesis

The major pathologic change is the increase of the number or the enlargement of the volume of adipose tissues. But the etiology is not completely clear, it may eventually be due to unequal metabolism of energy in the body, namely, more intake and less consumption, thus resulting in an abnormal level of body weight and bodily fat.

The factors that induce obesity in childhood mainly consist of three aspects such as parental obesity, neonatal overweight, breast feeding etc.. To control the neonatal body weight is the principal link of reducing fatness. Those who were fat in their infancies may also be fat in their adults, which account for 45% of the total. For those who are known as life-long obesity, the effect of reducing fatness among them is, in general, not ideal.

Adult obesity denotes those who become fat after the age of twenty. The major change among them is hypertrophies of the adipose cells, but the number of these cells does not increase, so that the effect on reducing fatness will be good.

Following the increase of age, obesity tends to aggravation. The incidence of obesity in patients over fifty years of age is as high as **40.3%**.

According to the TCM lore, the basic mechanism of this affection is deficiency of qi, and phlegm-turbidity is the product of pathology. Deficiency of Qi is closely related to the spleen and kidney. Weakness or disorder of spleen and kidney is the pathologic base of obesity.

Differentiation and Treatment of Common Syndromes

1. Type of humidity in spleen and turbid phlegm

Main Symptoms and Signs: Fat constitution, stiffness of chest and suffocation, shortness of breath and lack of strength, heaviness sensation of the body, lassitude, vertigo, palpitation, abdominal distention, scant food intake, sometimes dropsies of lower limbs, white or white greasy fur, slender or slender slippery pulse.

Recipe:

Folium Nelumbinis	12 g
Rhizoma Atractylodis Macrocephalae	12 g
Rhizoma Alismatis	15 g
Poria	15 g
Semen Cassiae	15 g
Semen Coicis	15 g
Radix Stephaniae	15 g
Pericarpium Citri Reticulatae	10 g

2. Type of excess heat in spleen and stomach

Main Symptoms and Signs: Polyphagia, obesity and robustness, liability to hunger, ruddy complexion, dry mouth and tongue, constipation (moving bowels once every two or three days, or even three to five days), red tongue proper with yellow thin fur, forceful taut pulse.

Recipe:

Radix Coptidis	10 g
Folium Cassiae	10 g

Radix et Rhizoma Rhei	10 g
Radix Rehmanniae	15 g
Prunellae Spica	12 g
Semen Cassiae	12 g

3. Type of Qi stagnancy and blood stasis

Main Symptom and Signs: Fat constitution, chest pain and flank distention, dysphoria and liability to anger, bulimia, irregular menstruation, or menopause, bias dry stool, dark purple tongue proper (with or without petechiae and/or ecchymoses), taut pulse.

Recipe:

Radix et Rhizoma Rhei	10 g
Resina Olibani	10 g
Pollen Typhae	10 g
Radix Ligustici Chuanxiong	12 g
Flos Carthami	12 g

Modification:

For lack of strength and shortness of breath severely in the above three types, Radix Astragali seu Hedysari or Radix Codonopsis Pilosulae 15 g are added. For dry mouth and tongue, Radix Ophiopogonis, Rhizoma Polygonati, at 10 g each are added. For dizziness and headache, Flos Chrysanthemi or Flos Chrysanthemi Indici 15 g are added. For rough urination, Herba Plantaginis 15 g, Polyporus Umbellatus 12 g are added. For severe phlegm − turbidity, Semen Pruni Armeniacae 10 g, Flos Rosae 10 g are added. For sore loins and weak knees, Fructus Ligustri Lucidi 15 g, Fructus Lycii 10 g are added.

Administration: One dose of the above drugs is decocted with water to be taken three times a day or the decoction is condensed to be taken 20 − 30 ml t. i. d.. One course of treatment consists of 15 − 45 days.

The above methods were used for treating 44 cases, of which 11 got marked effect (25.0%), 24 were effective (54.5%), with a total effective rate of 79.5%.

Simple Recipes and Proved Recipes

1. Reducing Lipid and Resisting Fat Tablets

Prescription: Reducing Lipid and Resisting Fat Tablets, i.e. Alcohol Extracted Rhubarb Tablets.

Administration: Tablets are taken at half of an hour before meals, 5 - 10 tablets b.i.d. It is appropriate to have the bowels moved once or twice a day after medication. Dosage can be modified according to the above stated requirement.

The above method was used in 64 cases, 26 got marked effect, the total effective rate amounted to 92.2%. At the same time, it was observed that the total hypotensive rate in 54 cases complicated with hypertension amounted to 88.9% The tablets have taken evident effect on patients of high cholesterol, high triglyceride, high lipoprotein B. 10 cases complicated with irregular menstruation restored normal.

2. Xiao - Pang Ling:

Recipe:

Semen Cassiae	30 g
Rhizoma Alismatis	15 g
Semen Pruni	15 g
Fructus Cinnabis	10 g
Fructus Crataegi	10 g

(2) Anti - Obesity Tea:

Folium Cassiae	10 g
Semen Persicae	10 g
Polyporus Umbellatus	10 g
Fructus Aurantii	10 g
Radix Astragali seu Hedysari	10 g

Administration: Xiao - Pang Ling is taken at one or two packets t.i.d. (weighing 20 g per packet) half of an hour before meals. Anti - Obesity Tea is infused with boiling water at 10 g b.i.d., t.i.d., or q.d.. A course of treatment consists of 30 days. In the period of treatment, diet should be controlled and appropriate exercises are advised.

The above methods were used for treating 96 cases. In the light of the observation of one treating course, the total effective rate accounted for 82.59%. At the same time, pantothen 0.2 g t.i.d. for 30 days was given to controls for contrast observation. And the total effective rate of them was only 43.3%. There existed very marked difference between the two groups ($P < 0.01$).

3. Lightening – Body Decoction

Recipe:

Herba Artemisiae Scopariae	40 g
Radix Polygoni Multiflori	20 g
Fructus Rosae Laevigatae	30 g
Rhizoma Polygonati	30 g
Fructus Crataegi	15 g
Radix Salviae Miltiorrhizae	20 g
Radix Puerariae	20 g
Radix et Rhizoma Rhei	10 g
Pulvis Notoginseng	5 g
Rhizoma Alismatis	5 g

Administration: The above drugs are decocted with water to be taken at one dose a day in two separate portions.

110 cases were treated with the above means, of which 47 got marked effect, 55 were effective, with a total effective rate of 92.7%. Observation was also performed among 54 patients with hyperlipemia. Of the 54, 19 got marked effect, 32 gained effectiveness, with a total effective rate of 94.9%.

4. Anti – Obesity and Reducing – Lipid Capsules

Recipe:

Radix Ginseng
Rhizoma Polygonati
Radix Polygoni Multiflori
Natrii Sulfas Exsiccatus
Semen Persicae

Administration: The above drugs are processed and made into capsules, each containing crude drug 0.5 g. Adults are given two or three capsules t.i.d.. A course of treatment consists of three months.

100 cases were treated with the above method. The effective rate was 96%. According to the observation, the capsules had no toxic side effect, Anti – obesity result might occur after the medication of 25 days. The effect grew evident subsequently. furthermore, the capsules had an ideal effectiveness in reducing fatness.

5. Jian Zhi Jian Fei Ling (Efficacious Remedy for Reducing Lipid and

Fatness)

Recipe:
> *Semen Cassia*
> *Fructus Crataegi*
> *Folium Camelliae Sinensis*

Administration: The above ingredients are prepared into oral solution to be taken t.i.d at 20 ml each time half of an hour before breakfast, lunch and supper. Those who had their body weight above 90 kg are advised to take ad extra dies of 20 ml before sleep.

100 cases were treated with the above method, of which 69 got marked effect, 23 were effective, with a total effective rate of 92%. As compared with the 100 controls given 20 mg of fenfluramine b.i.d. or t.i.d. at a total effective rate of 89%, the result was of marked significance ($P<0.05$).

6. Anti-Obesity Mixture

Recipe:

Powder for Gold Limb	18 g
Ramulus Sesami Indici	60 g
Cortex Paulowniae Fortunei	15 g
Exocarpium Citri Grandis	5 g
Poria	9 g
Rhizoma Alismatis	9 g

Administration: The above drugs are boiled in water to be taken twice a day at 30–60 ml each time. One course of treatment consists of one month.

90 cases were treated with the above method, of which 10 were cured, 24 got marked effect, 42 improved, with a total effective rate of 84.5%. Combined therapy of reducing fat and facilitating urination was performed for contrast observation among 42 cases, the effective rate was 59.3%. The difference between both groups was very marked.

Convenient Recipe

Recipe 1:

astragalus root	15 g
tetrandra root	15 g
white atractylodes rhizome	15 g
Chuanxiong rhizome	15 g

Simple Obesity

prepared fleece – flower root	15 g
oriental water plantain rhizome	30 g
raw hawthorn fruit	30 g
red sage root	30 g
oriental wormwood	30 g
waterbuffalo horn	30 g
epimedium	10 g
raw rhubarb	9 g

The above ingredients are boiled in water for 100 ml of decoction. 50 ml of decoction is taken orally each time, twice a day. For those with 25% over-weight, 150% of dosages, i.e. 150 ml, can be taken every day and can be taken in three times.

Recipe 2:

wolfberry fruit	9 g
fleece – flower root	15 g
cassia seed	15 g
hawthorn fruit	15 g
red sage root	20 g

The above ingredients are boiled in water for 1500 ml of decoction to drink as tea.

Recipe 3:

areca seed	30 g
magnolia bark	15 g
wine – fried rhubarb	9 g
green tangerine peel	15 g
atractylodes rhizome	15 g
pinellia tuber	15 g
poria	15 g
citron or trifoliate orange fruit	15 g
white mustard seed	9 g
burnt hawthorn fruit	15 g

All above drugs are to be decocted in water, for oral administration.

Recipe 4:

seaweed	15 g

prunella spike	15 g
coix seed	30 g
white mustard seed	9 g
hawthorn fruit	15 g
oriental water plantain rhizome	12 g
oriental wormwood	15 g
bupleurum root	9 g
licorice	6 g

All above drugs are to be decocted in water, for oral administration.

Patent Medicine

1. Ninghong Healthcare Tea (Ninghong Baojian Cha). Drink one bag each time, twice a day, and drink after mixed in water.

2. Seven Elimination Pills (Qi Xiao Wan). Take two pills a day, one in the morning and one in the evening respectively. Take before meals with warm water.

3. Wild – Goose Body – weight Reduction Tea (Dayan Jianfei Cha). Take one bag each time, three times a day, after mixed in water.

4. Rhubarb Tablets (Dahuang Pian). Take 5 tablets each time, three times a day, with warm water.

Acupuncture and Moxibustion

1. Body Acupuncture

Main Points: **Liángqiū (ST34)**, **Gōngsūn (SP4)**, **Qūchí (LI11)**, and **Xuèhǎi (SP10)**.

Complementary Points: Add **Nèitíng (ST44)** for excessive appetite; add **Tiānshū (ST25)** and **Zhīgōu (SJ6)** for constipation; add **Shuǐfēn (RN9)** and **Yīnlíngquán (SP9)** for scanty urine.

Method: All the above points are punctured with reduction. After the patient has the sore and distending sensation in the treatment, the needles can be manipulated repeatedly with light thrusting and heavy lifting and high-frequency twisting movement in large amplitude till the strong needling sensation occurs and within the tolerance of the patient.

2. Ear Acupuncture

Prescribed Points: Lung, Spleen, Large Intestine, and Sanjiao (Triple Energizer).

Simple Obesity

Method: After the skin of the auricular points is cleaned with alcohol cotton ball, the vaccaria seed is stuck on the center of a plaster in 0.8 cm^2, and then it can be pressed and stuck on the selected point. Every time in the hungry sensation, the herbal seed can be pressed for 5 minutes by the patient himself till there is a slight pain.

3. Acupuncture combined with ear point pressing with vegetable seeds

Selection of points: (1) Body points: **Liángqiū(ST34), Gōngsūn(SP4)**.

(2) Ear points: Mouth, Stomach, Spleen, Large Intestine, Intertragus, Triple Burner, Lung, Shenmen, Brain, Hunger Spot.

Manipulation: One body point is selected in each treatment to be punctured alternately with sedative maneuver. After gaining of sensation, needle is thrust gently and lifted heavily in rotations of big range and rapid frequency to enable the patient having an intense needling sensation. Later, G 6805 stimulator is connected by using a continuous wave. The capacity of the current is subject to the tolerance of the patient. The needle is retained for twenty minutes. After withdrawal of the needle, an intradermal pin at the style of a wheat grain is inserted at the depth of about 1 cm beneath the skin (the needle body is in vertical position with the circulation of the meridians), and then is fixed with a piece of adhesive plaster for two or three days. Five or six ear points are selected for use. A grain of cassia seed is adhered to the tender spot of the ear point region. Ear points at one side are used in one treatment. Both ears are used alternately. The patient is instructed to press the ear points and the intradermal needles twice or three times a day, at one or two minutes each time (per point). At the time of feeling hungry, or ten minutes before meals, to knead the points intensely is advised.

Treatment is given every other day or every three days. A course of treatment consists of ten treatments.

The above methods were used in treating 284 cases, of which 96 got marked effect, 150 gained effectiveness, with a total effective rate of 86.62%.

4. Plastering of cowbasil seed to treat obesity caused by endocrine disturbance

Ear points: Endocrine, Subcortex, Suppanene, Kidney, Triple Burner, Hunger Spot, Thirst Spot are selected. For somnolence, ear point Sympathy is added. For female patients, ear point Ovary is added. Cow－basil seed is fixed on the ear point with a piece of adhesive plaster for two days. Twenty days consisted of a course. Both ears are stimulated alternately. The next course starts after an interval of five days.

460 cases were treated with this method for a period of three courses. Result: 387 cases gained marked effect, 61 cases gained effectiveness, with a total effective rate of 97.4%. In the duration of treatment, patients were instructed to eat more vegetables and fruit, and to eat less high－fat or high calory food for the sake of enhancing curative effects. (Patients of this group were all foreigners.)

5. Acupuncture and cupping

Selection of points:

Group I: **Zhōngwǎn (RN12), Tiānshū (ST25), Guānyuán (RN4), Zúsānlǐ (ST36), Yīnlíngquán(SP9)**.

Group II: **Jùquè (RN14), Dàhéng (SP15), Qìhǎi (RN6), Fēnglóng (ST40), Sānyīnjiāo(SP6)**.

Manipulations: The above points are pierced and cupped with the exception of **Zúsānlǐ(ST36), Yīnlíngquán(SP9), Fēnglóng(ST40)** and **Sānyīnjiāo(SP6)** upon which only acupuncture is used. Two groups of points are stimulated alternately. For patients with big hip, **Jīmén(SP11), Bìguān(ST31)** can be added. All the points are subject to sedative maneuver, that is, to apply light thrust and heavy lift repeatedly with rotations of big range and rapid frequency. Needles are retained in situ for thirty minutes. After withdrawal of the needle, points at the abdominal region are given an extra cupping of fifteen minutes. Treatment is given once a day. Ten days consisted of a course of treatment. Four courses are required. Between each course, an interval of three days is advised.

80 cases were treated with the above methods. Of them 24 got short－term clinical cure, 14 got marked effect, 31 gained effectiveness, with a total effective rate of 86.25%.

6. Jian Mei Ling (Efficacious Remedy for Health and Beauty)

Administration: (1) Group of Jian Mei Ling plus Auto－massaging: Hot compression with towel is first used, then about 5g of Jian Mei Ling is evenly coated on the abdomen with both hands massaging the belly toward the ipsilateral groin from upper side to lower side for thirty minutes. When Jian Mei

Simple Obesity

Long turned from yellow color into milky white or even transparent color, it is totally absorbed by the slim of the belly. Treatment is given once a day. Ten treatments consisted of one course. (2) Group of Jian Mei Ling plus callisthenic device: HP - Qigong frequency spectrum radiation imitator is used at the voltage of 200v ± 10%, the frequency of 50 - 60 Hz, the power of 250 - 300 w or YHD infrared therapeutic lamp is used. The patients are instructed to lie in supine position with their abdomen exposed. The imitator is directed to point **Qìhăi(RN6)**. The distance between the imitator and abdomen is about 25 - 30 cm, and it is appropriate for the patients to have a warm feeling. When the local part shows a reticular erythema, about 5 g of natural Jian Mei Ling is coated on the abdomen, and massaged with the same method described before. Then DJ - 1 callisthenic device is used for 20 - 30 minutes, once a day. The days consisted of a course of treatment.

After ten treatments, in the first group of thirty cases, 8 got special effect, 10 got marked effect and 11 got effectiveness. In the second group of forty cases, 30 got special effect, 8 got marked effect and 2 got effectiveness. The difference between the two groups is very marked ($P<0.001$).

Qigong

Preparation: One hand is put on the chest. The other hand is put on the abdomen.

Strength Direction: The chest is straightened and the abdomen is held in the inhalation. The chest is contracted and the abdomen is straightened in the exhalation. The abdomen is requested to be straightened to the utmost when the chest is contracted and the abdomen is straightened. To practice the exercise for 40 times before three meals every day can mostly eliminate the hungry sensation. If the hungry sensation still exists, it is advisable to practice the exercise for 20 times more.

After the practice of the exercise, it is possible to decrease the food intake naturally, but the symptoms of dizziness, lassitude caused by glycopenia should be avoided.

2. Manipulation: Rejuvenescence Prowess (inner cultivating prowess of Taoists for life preservation and longevity) includes tri - ring prowess, that is mutual help and check of heart and kidney (back and forth ring prowess), mu-

tual return of yin and yang (right and left ring prowess), transformation of wu xing or namely five elements (upper and lower ring prowess).

(1) Rejuvenescence Prowess includes visualization of youth, beginning posture of Daoyin, hiding Qi and nursing spirits, shivering prowess and gentle conclusion.

(2) Roving dragon Prowess. The tri-ring prowess is to be practiced at half of an hour before supper for fifteen minutes. The rejuvenescence prowess and the roving dragon prowess are practiced in the morning or before sleep for fifteen minutes.

42 cases were treated with this method. According to the observation of three months, 15% of the total their body weight reduced, 95% had their waist circumference reduced.

Massage

The patient is asked to lie on the back, The chest, abdomen and two lower limbs can be kneaded. **Qūchí(LI11), Yángchí(SJ4), Zhōngwǎn(RN12), Zúsānlǐ(ST36), and Tàixī(KI3)** are pressed and **Guānyuán(RN4)** is grasped. Then the patient turns to lie on the stomach. The back, waist and posterior aspects of the lower limbs are kneaded with **Shēnzhù(DU12)** and **Géshū(BL17)** pressed. Each of the above points is pressed for one minute. **Guānyuán(RN4)** is emphatically grasped for 3-5 minutes.

Medicated Diet

1. 300 grams of wax gourd and some dried shrimp shells are boiled and seasoned as soup.

2. The external peel of watermelon is boiled in water to be taken as tea.

3. Frequent intake of dressed cucumber.

Chapter Nine
Bromhidrosis

Bromhidrosis refers to foul-smelling sweat from axillary space or other parts of the body. The patient should be given diet nursing in combination with effective treatment.

External Treatment

    Recipe: *Zhi huchou fang*

Flos Magnoliae	2 g
Rhizoma Ligustici Chuanxiong	2 g
Herba Asari	2 g
Wildginger	2 g
Rhizoma Ligustici	2 g

Soak the above ingredients in 20 ml of white spirit and 10 ml of edible vinegar for 12 hours. Clean the axillae up and apply the tincture on both sides at bedtime. *Flos Magnoliae*, *Rhizoma Ligustici Chuanxiong*, *Rhizoma Ligustici* can disperse wind evil and dissolve dampness stagnation, regulate qi and blood circulation. *Wildginger* is so fragrant that can conceal the foul-smelling sweat. Acrid food prohibited during the course of treatment.

    Recipe: *Tuoseng fen*

litharge	3 g

Grind litharge into fine powder and apply it on the axilla. Clean it 10 minutes later. Oral administration prohibited!

    Recipe: *Shihui san fang*

Calx	200 g

Radix Aucklandiae	60 g
Resin of sweetgum	60 g
Actinoliti	60 g
Pericarpium Citri Reticulatae	60 g
Alum	120 g

Stir-fry the ingredients until they are done. Grind them into fine powder and wrap it in a piece of gauze. Clean the axilla up and place the medicated gauze parcel in it. Adduct the upper arm to clamp the parcel for one hour.

Recipe: *Zhi yechou fang*

Calium Hydroxide	100 g
Herba Portulacae	60 g
Alum	90 g
Rhizoma Nardostachyos	30 g

Grind the above drugs into fine powder. Wipe the affected part with a piece of gauze until it is congested. Apply the powder on it.

Internal Treatment

Recipe: *Zhi shentichou ling xiang fang*

Moschus	1 g
Ligni Aquilariae	1 g
Lignum Santali Albi	1 g
Borneolum Syntheticum	1 g
Flos Caryophylli	15 g
Caryophylli	15 g
Rhizoma Nardostachyos	15 g
Rhizoma Cimicifugae	2 g
Tulipa Gesneriana	2 g
chicken-bone herb	15 g

Grind the above drugs into fine powder and make it into honeyed pills. Each weighs about 3 g. Take 3 pills with salt water on an empty stomach. Contraindicated for cases with syndrome of *yin*-deficiency and *blood*-heat.

Bromhidrosis

Recipe: Shi xiang yuan

Ligni Aquilariae	30 g
Moschus	30 g
Lignum Santali Albi	30 g
Radix Aucklandiae	30 g
Melilotus Officinalis	30 g
Radix Angelicae Dahuricae	30 g
Lophanthus Rugosus	30 g
Rhizoma Nardostachyos	30 g
Herba Asari	30 g
Rhizoma Ligustici Chuanxiong	30 g
Semen Arecae	30 g
Fructus Amomi Rotundus	30 g
Rhizoma Cyperi	15 g
Flos Caryophylli	2 g

Grind the above drugs into fine powder and make it into honeyed pills. Each weighs about 1 g. Take one pill in the mouth and swallow the dissolved. Acrid food prohibited. It is not suitable for long-term administration. Contraindicated for cases with syndrome of hyperactivity due to *yin*-deficiency.

Recipe: Xiang shen wan

Fructus Amomi Rotundus	120 g
Radix Aucklandiae	60 g
Lignum Santali Albi	30 g
Rhizoma Nardostachyos	30 g
Melilotus Officinalis	45 g
Flos Caryophylli	25 g
Radix Angelicae Dahuricae	15 g
Radix Angelicae Sinensis	15 g
Radix Aconiti Praeparata	15 g
Semen Arecae	15 g
Kaempferia Galanga	15 g
Radix Glycyrrhizae Praeparata	15 g
Fructus Alpiniae Oxyphyllae	15 g

Cortex Cinnamomi	15 g
Moschus	1 g

Grind the above drugs into fine powder and make it into honeyed pills. Each weighs about 1 g. Take pill in the mouth and swallow it when it is dissolved. It is not suitable for long-term administration. Contraindicated for cases with syndrome of hyperactivity due to *yin*-deficiency.

Recipe: *Xiang shen fang*

Semen Benincase	2 g
Rhizoma Ligustici Chuanxiong	2 g
Rhizoma Ligustici	2 g
wildginger	2 g
Radix Angelicae Sinensis	2 g
Herba Asari	2 g
Radix Ledebouriellae	2 g

Grind the above drugs into fine powder and take it orally, three times daily.

Chapter Ten
Seborrheic Dermatitis

Seborrheic dermatitis is call *"baixie feng"* in traditional Chinese medicine. It is caused by wind attack in hair and scalp in combination with asthenic heat due to *yin*-deficiency resulting in blood-dryness which leads to malnutrition of scalp. Treatment principles such as strenthenging superficies, dispersing wind-heat, clearing away blood-heat and moisturizing dryness are performed respectively or combinatively according to the condition of the patient.

External Treatment

Recipe: *Mutou tang fang*
Semen Cannabis	150 g
Radix Gentianae Macrophyllae	150 g
Fructus Gleditsiae	150 g

Grind the ingredients into powder and soak it in water for 12 hours. Remove the dregs and heat the medicated water until it is warm enough for washing hair.

Semen Cannabis has the effect of moisturizing dryness, dispersing wind evil, relieving itching. *Radix Gentianae Macrophyllae* can warm collaterals of the superficies and relieve superficial syndrome caused by wind attack. *Fructus Gleditsiae* is effective for removing dirt.

Recipe: *Toufeng baixie fang*
Fructus Viticis	120 g
Radix Ledebouriellae	90 g
Ramulus Loranthis	90 g

Radix Gentianae Macrophyllae	30 g
Semen Cannabis	120 g
Radix Angelicae Dahuricae	120 g

Decoct the above ingredients in 4 liters of water until 3 liters of filtered decoction retained. Wash hair with the decoction.

Fructus Viticis, *Radix Ledebouriellae* and *Radix Angelicae Dahuricae* eliminate wind evil in the upper energizer. *Ramulus Loranthis* and *Semen Cannabis* moisturize dryness of the viscera in order to prevent the occurring of internal wind due to blood dryness resulting from *yin*-deficiency. *Radix Gentianae Macrophyllae* can warm collaterals of the superficies and relieve superficial syndrome caused by wind attack. Add 100 g of *Natrii Sulphas* in case of severe wind-heat attack.

Recipe: Zhiyi xi fang

Frucus Xanthii	30 g
Semen Vaccariae	30 g
Radix Sophorae Flavescentis	15 g
Alumen	9 g

Decoct the ingredients for washing scalp. Once every three days.

Frucus Xanthii has the effect of dissolving dampness, dispersing wind. *Semen Vaccariae* is able to promote blood circulation and disperse stagnation. *Radix Sophorae Flavescentis* can clear away heat-toxin and eliminate dampness. *Alumen* can dry the dampness and restrain seborrhea. The prescription is effective for cases with severe seborrhea.

Internal Treatment

Recipe: Fangfeng jingjie san

Herba Schizonepetae	240 g
Rhizoma Atractylodis	240 g
Radix Glycyrrhizae Praeparata	105 g
Flos Chrysanthemi	15 g
Rhizoma Ligustici Chuanxiong	90 g
Radix Angelicae Dahuricae	90 g

Rhizoma seu Radix Notopterygii	90 g
Radix Ledebouriellae	90 g

Grind the above drugs into fine powder and make it into honeyed pills. Each weighs about 1 g. Take one pill each time. For the case of deficiency type, *Radix Astragali seu Hedysari* 24 g, *Rhizoma Atractylodis Macrocephalae* 9 g, *Radix Ledebouriellae* should be added.

Recipe: Qufeng huanji wan

Semen Sesami	60 g
Rhizoma Atractylodis	60 g
Rhizoma Achyranthis Bidentatae	60 g
Rhizoma Acori Graminei	60 g
Radix Sophorae Flavescentis	60 g
Radix Polygoni Multiflori	60 g
Radix Trichosanthis	60 g
Radix Clematidis	60 g
Radix Angelicae Sinensis	30 g
Rhizoma Ligustici Chuanxiong	30 g
Radix Glycyrrhizae	30 g

Grind the above drugs into fine powder and make it into honeyed pills. Each weighs about 1 g. Take 9 pills each time.

The prescription is most effective for cases with long-term seborrheic dermatitis manifesting syndrome of wind-heat stagnation in the scalp. *Semen Sesami*, *Rhizoma Achyranthis Bidentatae*, *Radix Polygoni Multiflori* and *Radix Angelicae Sinensis* invigorate kidney-yin and liver-yin to eliminate *blood*-dryness; *Radix Trichosanthis* can moisturize dryness of tissues; *Rhizoma Atractylodis*, *Radix Sophorae Flavescentis*, *Rhizoma Acori Calami*, *Radix Clematidis* and *Rhizoma Ligustici Chuanxiong* etc. disperse wind evil.

Chapter Eleven
Xerosis Pilorum

Xerosis pilorum is usually caused by insufficiency of both *qi* and *blood* resulting in malnutrition of hair. Treatment principle of invigorating *qi* and *blood* in combination with moisturizing xerosis is performed.

External Treatment

    Recipe: *Sanggen baiye tang*

Cortex Mori Radicis	480 g
Cacumen Biotae	480 g

All the above drugs decocted in 3 liters of water until it comes to boil. Wash hair with the warm decoction. The drugs have the effect of clearing away heat and moisturizing dryness.

    Recipe: *Changfa runze fang*

Fructus Mori	30 g
Flos Gardeniae	30 g
Pericarpium Granati	30 g
Fructus Chebulae	30 g
Herba Nelumbinis	30 g
Herba Asari	30 g
Radix Angelicae Dahuricae	15 g
Rhizoma Ligustici	30 g
Melilotus Officinalis	30 g
Radix Ampelopsis	30 g
Natrii Sulphas	30 g

Cortex Lycii Radicis	30 g
Gallae Turcicae	30 g

Grind the above drugs into fine powder and wrap it with a piece of gauze. Soak the gauze bag in millet wine in a sealed jar for 49 days. Comb hair after applying the medicated wine on hair.

This prescription is effective for cases with severe wind-heat syndrome.

Internal Treatment

Recipe: *Qinjiao wan*

Pericarpium Zanthoxyli	30 g
Radix Rehmanniae	30 g
Flos Inulae	30 g
Radix Angelicae Dahuricae	30 g

Grind the above drugs into fine powder and make it into honeyed pills. Each weighs about 1 g. Take 30 pills with millet wine each time. This prescription is most effective for cases with *yang*-deficiency. *Pericarpium Zanthoxyli* can warm the middle-jiao to disperse cold, promote blood circulation to nourish hair. *Radix Angelicae Dahuricae* alleviates itching. *Radix Rehmanniae* invigorates *blood* to nourish hair.

Recipe: *Digupi wan*

Cortex Lycii Radicis	150 g
Radix Rehmanniae	150 g
Rhizoma Achyranthis Bidentatae	90 g
Fructus Rubi	90 g
Radix Astragali seu Hedysari	90 g
Fructus Schisandrae	90 g
Semen Persicae	120 g
Semen Cuscutae	120 g
Fructus Tribuli	120 g

Grind the above drugs into fine powder and make it into honeyed pills. Each weighs about 1 g. Take 40 pills with warm millet wine on an empty stomach.

The prescription is most effective for cases with *yin*-deficiency. *Cortex Lycii Radicis*, *Radix Rehmanniae*, *Rhizoma Achyranthis Bidentatae*, *Fructus Schisandrae*, *Semen Cuscutae* etc. invigorate *yin-blood* of the liver and kidney. *Radix Astragali seu Hedysari* and *Fructus Rubi* enhance *qi* of the lung and kidney. *Semen Persicae* and *Fructus Tribuli* disperse *qi* stagnation and remove blood-stasis to nourish hair.

Chapter Twelve
Achromotrichia

Achromotrichia is usually caused by malnutrition of hair due to deficiency of qi and blood and insufficiency of liver-yin and kidney-yin. Invigorating drugs are generally used.

External Treatment

Recipe: Dingxiang zhu san

Caryophylli	3 g
Gallae Turcicae	3 g
Rhizoma Nardostachyos	30 g
Fructus Amomi	4.5 g
Rhizoma Bletillae	8 g
Fructus Chebulae	6 g
Kaempferia Galanga	3 g

Decoct the above ingredients in 300 ml of water until 200 ml of filtered decoction retained. Apply the decoction on hair at bedtime and wash hair with clean water the next morning.

Recipe: Moding heifa fang

Radix Angelicae Dahuricae	30 g
Radix Aconiti Praeparata	30 g
Fructus Forsythiae	30 g
Radix Ledebouriellae	30 g
Cacumen Biotae	30 g
Melilotus Officinalis	30 g

    Fructus Viticis   30 g
    Natrii Sulphas   30 g

Grind the above drugs into powder and soak it in 1,000 ml of millet wine for three days. Apply a right amount of medicated wine on hair and scalp. Rubbing manipulation required.

Recipe: Zelan jian
    Herba Asari   60 g
    Radix Dipsaci   60 g
    Fructus Gleditsiae   60 g
    Ramulus Wallichii seu Puberulii   60 g
    Herba Lycopi   60 g
    Cortex Magnoliae Officinalis   60 g
    Radix Aconiti   60 g
    Illicii Anisati   60 g
    Rhizoma Atractylodis Macrocephalae   60 g
    Pericarpium Zanthoxyli   60 g
    Semen Armeniacae Amarum   45 g

Soak the ingredients in white spirit for 12 hours. Decoct the tincture and dregs until it is done. Wash hair with the decoction at bedtime. Clean hair with pure water the next morning.

In the prescription, *Pericarpium Zanthoxyli*, *Radix Aconiti* and *Herba Asari* disperse coldness in the meridians and collateral. *Ramulus Wallichii seu Puberulii* and *Illicium Anisatum* disperse wind-evil. *Semen Armeniacae Amarum*, *Cortex Magnoliae Officinalis* and *Rhizoma Atractylodis Macrocephalae* promote qi circulation and eliminate dampness. *Herba Lycopi*, *Radix Dipsaci* and *Fructus Gleditsiae* promote *blood* circulation and remove *blood*-deficiency. It is effective for cases with stagnation of wind, coldness and phlegm-dampness evil in hair roots, stagnating the transportation of *qi* and *blood* leading to malnutrition of hair.

Recipe: Shen zhen fa
    Rhizoma Ligustici Chuanxiong   30 g
    Radix Platycodi   30 g

Achromotrichia

Radix Cynanchi Atrati	30 g
Herba Schizonepetae	30 g
Flos Magnoliae	30 g
wildginger	30 g
Rhizoma Atractylodis Macrocephalae	30 g
Rhizoma Ligustici	30 g
Pericarpium Zanthoxyli	30 g
Cortex Cinnamomi	30 g
Rhizoma Zingiberis	30 g
Radix Ledebouriellae	30 g
Radix Ginseng	30 g
Radix Angelicae Sinensis	30 g
Radix Angelicae Dahuricae	30 g
Herba Cistanchis	30 g
Semen Biotae	30 g
Semen Coicis	30 g
Flos Farfarae	30 g
Radix Gentianae Macrophyllae	30 g
Radix Aconiti	30 g
Radix Aconiti Praeparata	30 g
Hellebore	30 g
Fructus Gleditsiae	30 g
Fructus Foeniculi	30 g
Rhizoma Pinelliae	30 g
Alumen	30 g
Herba Asari	30 g

Grind the above drugs into powder. Fill a pillow with the powder. Sleep with the head on the medicated pillow.

Recipe: *Qingsi san*

Radix Angelicae Dahuricae	9 g
Poria	9 g
Radix Angelicae Sinensis	9 g
Rhizoma Ligustici Chuanxiong	9 g

Radix Glycyrrhizae	9 g
Herba Asari	15 g
Radix Polygoni Multiflori	15 g
Gypsum Lamelliforme	15 g
Rhizoma Cimicifugae	6 g
Radix Rehmanniae	6 g
Cortex Lycii Radicis	6 g
Flos Caryophylli	9 g

Grind the drugs into fine powder and brush teeth with it, twice daily.

According to the theory of traditional Chinese medicine, there is special relation between hair and bones (teeth), which are all controlled by kidney-qi. In the prescription, *Rhizoma Cimicifugae*, *Gypsum Lamelliforme*, *Radix Angelicae Sinensis*, *Rhizoma Ligustici Chuanxiong*, *Herba Asari* strengthen teeth to promote the function of kidney-qi in a special way. *Radix Angelicae Dahuricae*, *Radix Polygoni Multiflori*, *Radix Rehmanniae*, *Poria*, *Cortex Lycii Radicis* and *Flos Caryophylli* nourish hair by invigorating kidney-qi.

Internal Treatment

Recipe: *Tusizi wan*

Semen Cuscutae	90 g
Cortex Lycii Radicis	90 g
Fructus Aurantii	240 g
Succus Cyathulae Radicis	300 ml
Succus Rehmanniae Radicis	300 ml

Grind the first three drugs into fine powder and mix it with juice of *Radix Rehmanniae* and *Radix Cyathulae*. Dry the mixture and make it into honeyed pills. Each weighs about 1 g. Take 15 pills with warm millet after breakfast.

In the prescription, *Radix Rehmanniae*, *Radix Cyathulae*, *Semen Cuscutae* and *Cortex Lycii Radicis* are effective for nourishing hair. *Fructus Aurantii* promotes qi circulation in order to increase the effectiveness.

Recipe: *Zhi fabai linghei fang*

Radix Rehmanniae	2.5 kg
Cortex Acanthopanacis Radicis	240 g
Rhizoma Achyranthis Bidentatae	240 g

Grind the above drugs into fine powder and take 9 g with warm millet wine on an empty stomach. The prescription has the effect of invigorating liver and kidney, enhancing *qi* and *blood* to promote the growth and nutrition of hair.

Recipe: *Shenxian xunlao dan*

Fructus Lycii	300 g
Radix Rehmanniae	150 g
Radix Rehmanniae Praeparata	150 g
Rhizoma Dioscoreae	150 g
Radix Polygoni Multiflori	0.6 kg
Pericarpium Zanthoxyli	90 g
Rhizoma Achyranthis Bidentatae	90 g
Semen Phaseoli	150 g
Herba Cistanchis	150 g
Rhizoma Ligustici	300 g

Grind the above drugs into fine powder and make it into honeyed pills. Each weighs about 1 g. Take 30 pills with salt water or warm millet wine on an empty stomach each time. This prescription is suitable for cases with grey hair due to insufficiency of kidney-essence.

Recipe: *Shenxian bulao dan*

Fructus Lycii	60 g
Semen Cuscutae	60 g
Rhizoma Acori Graminei	30 g
Semen Biotae	30 g
Radix Cyathulae	45 g
Cortex Eucommiae	45 g
Cortex Lycii Radicis	30 g
Radix Rehmanniae	60 g

Radix Angelicae Sinensis	60 g
Radix Codonopsis Pilosulae	60 g
Radix Morindae Officinalis	30 g

Grind the above drugs into fine powder and make it into honeyed pills. Each weighs about 1 g. Take 70 pills with salt water or warm millet wine on an empty stomach each time. This prescription is suitable for cases with grey hair due to insufficiency of both kidney-essence and kidney-*yang*.

Recipe: *Wushen huantong dan*

Lapis Rubri	180 g
Pericarpium Zanthoxyli	90 g
Cinnabaris	15 g
Poria	120 g
Olibani	30 g
Fructus Ziziphi Jujubae	a right amount

Grind the above drugs into fine powder and make it into honeyed pills. Each weighs about 1 g. Take 30 pills on an empty stomach. This prescription is effective for cases with grey hair due to blood-stasis in the heart meridian resulting in malnutrition of hair.

Dietetic Treatment

Name:

brown sugar	500 g
Semen Juglandis	250 g
Semen Sesami	250 g

Stir-fry walnut kernel and sesame seed until it is done. Cook brown sugar with a small amount of water until it is dissolved. Add walnut kernel and sesame seed in it and mix it well. Take a right amount of the medicated sugar daily.

Name: *Wufa migao*

Radix Polygoni Multiflori	200 g
Poria	200 g

Radix Angelicae Sinensis	50 g
Fructus Lycii	50 g
Semen Cuscutae	50 g
Rhizoma Achyranthis Bidentatae	50 g
Fructus Psoraleae	50 g
Semen Sesami	50 g

Soak the drugs in a right amount of water for one hour. Then decoct them over a slow fire for one hour. Filter the decoction and continue decocting the dregs with a right amount of water. Repeat the progress of decocting and filtering again. Then mix the flitered decoction together and cook it over a slow fire until it is extracted enough. Add honey (same amount as the extracted decoction) in the extract and stir it well, cook it until it comes to boil. Store it in a chinese jar for later oral administration.

Chapter Thirteen
Halitosis

Halitosis here refers to foul breath from mouth and is not secondary to other known diseases.

External Treatment

Recipe: *Huoxiang yin*
    Lophanthus Rugosus   a right amount
Wash the drug clean and decoct it to make gargle.

Recipe: *Chuanxiong hanshu fang*
    Rhizoma Ligustici Chuanxiong   a right amount
Decoct the drug and filter the decoction to make gargle.

Recipe: *Xiongqiong tang*

Rhizoma Ligustici Chuanxiong	90 g
Radix Angelicae Sinensis	90 g
Radix Angelicae Pubescentis	120 g
Herba Asari	120 g
Radix Angelicae Dahuricae	120 g

Decoct the drugs and filter the decoction to make gargle.

Recipe: *Huatuo zhichou fang*
    Radix Sophorae Flavescentis   a right amount
Decoct the drug and filter the decoction to make gargle.

Halitosis

Recipe: *Shengma san*

Rhizoma Cimicifugae	60 g
Radix Ledebouriellae	30 g
Radix Angelicae Sinensis	15 g
Radix Angelicae Dahuricae	15 g
Rhizoma Ligustici Chuanxiong	6 g
Rhizoma Ligustici	6 g
Moschus	1 g
Radix Glycyrrhizae	15 g
Radix Aucklandiae	2 g
Herba Asari	2 g

Grind the above drugs into fine powder and apply 6 g on the gingivae each time.

Recipe: *Xiangru yin*

Herba Elsholtziae seu Moslae

Decoct the drug and filter the decoction to make gargle.

Recipe: *Xixin yin*

Herba Asari	a right amount

Decoct the drug and filter the decoction to make gargle.

Internal Treatment

Recipe: *Wuxiang wan*

Fructus Amomi Rotundus	30 g
Flos Caryophylli	30 g
Lophanthus Rugosus	30 g
Melilotus Officinalis	30 g
Radix Aucklandiae	30 g
Radix Angelicae Dahuricae	30 g
Cortex Cinnamomi	30 g
Rhizoma Cyperi	60 g
Rhizoma Nardostachyos	15 g

Radix Angelicae Sinensis	15 g
Semen Arecae	10 g

Grind the above drugs into fine powder and make it into honeyed pills. Each weighs about 1 g. Take one pill in mouth and swallow the dissolved.

Recipe: **Dingxiang wan**

Flos Caryophylli	9 g
Radix Glycyrrhizae Praeparata	3 g
Rhizoma Ligustici Chuanxiong	6 g
Radix Angelicae Dahuricae	2 g

Grind the above drugs into fine powder and make it into honeyed pill. Take the pill in mouth and swallow the dissolved.

Recipe: **Fujian xiangcha bing**

Ligni Aquilariae	30 g
Lignum Santali Albi	30 g
catechu	60 g
Radix Glycyrrhizae	15 g
Moschus	1 g
Borneolum Syntheticum	1 g

Grind the above drugs into fine powder and make it into honeyed pills. Each weighs about 1 g. Take one pill in mouth and swallow the saliva.

Recipe: **Qing qi wan**

Pericarpium Citri Reticulatae Viride	15 g
Rhizoma Coptidis	15 g
Radix Scutellariae	15 g
Radix Glycyrrhizae	15 g
Gypsum Fibrosum	30 g
Lignum Santali Albi	30 g

Grind the above drugs into fine powder and make it into honeyed pills. Each weighs about 1 g. Take one pill each time. Contraindicated for cases with deficiency of the spleen and stomach.

Halitosis

Acupuncture and Moxibustion

1. Apply three moxa cones on the point **Láogōng(PC8)** respectively. Effective for foul breath due to heat evil stagnating in the heart meridian.

Puncture **Dàlíng(PC7)** for 0.3 to 0.5 cun. It is effective for foul breath due to heat evil stagnating in the heart meridian.

Chapter Fourteen
Hygiene of Oral Cavity

Prescriptions introduced here are effective for cleaning oral cavity and protecting teeth, preventing oral diseases.

Recipe:

Gypsum Fibrosum	6 g
Herba Menthae	3 g
Pericarpium Zanthoxyli	3 g
Cortex Moutan Radicis	6 g
Radix Angelicae Pubescentis	6 g
edible salt	6 g

Decoct the ingredients and filter the decoction to make gargle.

Recipe: Kaichi fangfeng san

Radix Ledebouriellae	2 g
Rhizoma Cimicifugae	2 g
Herba Asari	2 g
Gypsum Lamelliforme	15 g
Cinnabaris	1 g
Ligni Aquilariae	1 g
Flos Caryophylli	1 g
Moschus	1 g

Grind the drugs into fine powder and brush teeth with the powder.

Recipe: Lanshi caji

Moschus	1 g

Hygiene of Oral Cavity

Radix Rehmanniae	2 g
Radix Stephaniae Tetrandrae	2 g
Radix Rehmanniae Praeparata	2 g
Radix Angelicae Sinensis	3 g
Radix Ginseng	3 g
Cortex Alpiniae Katsumadai Semen	3 g
Rhizoma Cimicifugae	4 g
Rhizoma Coptidis	6 g
Fructus Amomi Rotundus	9 g
Semen Alpiniae Katsumadai	9 g
Gallae Turcicae	10 g
Galla Chinensis	5 g

Grind the above drugs into fine powder. Gargle oral cavity with warm water. Then brush teeth with a right amount of the powder.

Recipe: Jili san

Fructus Tribuli	30 g
Herba Asari	5 g
Rhizoma Ligustici Chuanxiong	5 g

Grind the above drugs into fine powder. Gargle oral cavity with warm water. Then brush teeth with a right amount of the powder.

Recipe: Laoya fang

Herba Schizonepetae
Rhizoma Ligustici Chuanxiong
Herba Asari
Radix Angelicae Sinensis

Grind the above drugs into fine powder. Gargle oral cavity with warm water. Then brush teeth with a right amount of the powder. Gargle mouth with warm water five minutes later. Effective for preventing odontoseisis.

Recipe: Guchi mifang

Radix et Rhizoma Rhei	30 g
Radix et Rhizoma Rhei Praeparata	30 g

Gypsum Fibrosum	30 g
Gypsum Fibrosi Praeparata	30 g
Rhizoma Drynariae	30 g
Cortex Eucommiae	30 g
edible salt	30 g
Alumen	15 g
Radix Angelicae Sinensis	15 g

Grind the above drugs into fine powder. Gargle oral cavity with warm water. Then brush teeth and gingiva with a right amount of the powder. Gargle mouth with warm water five minutes later. Effective for odontalgia due to hyperactivity of stomach-*fire*, also for preventing odontoseisis and gingivitis.

Recipe: Guchi liangfang

Edible salt	15 g
Gypsum Fibrosum	15 g
Fructus Psoraleae	12 g
Pericarpium Zanthoxyli	5 g
Radix Angelicae Dahuricae	5 g
Radix Ledebouriellae	8 g
Herba Menthae	8 g
Herba Ecliptae	8 g
Herba Asari	5 g

Dry the above drugs in the sun and grind them into fine powder. Gargle oral cavity with warm water. Then brush teeth and gingiva with a right amount of the powder. Gargle mouth with warm water five minutes later. Effective for odontoseisis.

Recipe: Chenxiyi yayao

Fructus Gleditsiae	60 g
Rhizoma Zingiberis Recens	60 g
Rhizoma Cimicifugae	60 g
Radix Rehmanniae Praeparata	60 g
Herba Ecliptae	60 g
Flos Sophorae	60 g

Hygiene of Oral Cavity

Herba Asari	60 g
Herba Nelumbinis	60 g
edible salt	60 g

Grind the above drugs into fine powder and heat it until it is slightly carbonized. Gargle oral cavity with warm water. Then brush teeth and gingiva with a right amount of the powder. Gargle mouth with warm water five minutes later. Effective for odontoseisis.

Recipe: *Wuxu guchi bushen san*

Radix Angelicae Sinensis	75 g
Rhizoma Ligustici Chuanxiong	75 g
Herba Schizonepetae	75 g
Rhizoma Cyperi	75 g
Radix Paeoniae Alba	75 g
Fructus Lycii	75 g
Radix Rehmanniae Praeparata	75 g
Radix Cyathulae	60 g
Herba Asari	9 g
Fructus Psoraleae	45 g
Rhizoma Cimicifugae	15 g
edible salt	90 g

Grind the above drugs into fine powder and make it into pills with cooked polished round-grained rice. Each weighs about 3 g. Take one pill in mouth and swallow the medicated saliva. Effective for odontoseisis.

Recipe: *Shengma kaichi fang*

Rhizoma Cimicifugae	15 g
Radix Angelicae Dahuricae	1 g
Rhizoma Ligustici	1 g
Herba Asari	1 g
Ligni Aquilariae	1 g
Gypsum Lamelliforme	2 g

Grind the above drugs into fine powder. Gargle oral cavity with warm water. Then brush teeth with a right amount of the powder. Gargle mouth with warm water five minutes later. Effective for cleaning teeth.

Recipe: *Yuqian jiechi san*

Gypsum Fibrosum	120 g
Rhizoma Cyperi	30 g
Radix Angelicae Dahuricae	22 g
Rhizoma Nardostachyos	4.5 g
Kaempferia Galanga	4.5 g
Lophanthus Rugosus	4.5 g
Ligni Aquilariae	4.5 g
Rhizoma Ligustici Chuanxiong	10 g
Melilotus Officinalis	10 g
Herba Asari	15 g
Radix Ledebouriellae	15 g

Grind the above drugs into fine powder. Gargle oral cavity with warm water. Then brush teeth with a right amount of the powder. Gargle mouth with warm water five minutes later. Effective for cleaning teeth.

Recipe: *Kaishi shigao san*

Gypsum Fibrosum	15 g
Gypsum Lamelliforme	15 g
Cinnabaris	15 g
Rhizoma Cimicifugae	15 g
Radix Angelicae Dahuricae	15 g
Herba Asari	15 g
Rhizoma Ligustici	15 g
Ligni Aquilariae	30 g
Moschus	1 g

Grind the above drugs into fine powder. Gargle oral cavity with warm water. Then brush teeth with a right amount of the powder. Gargle mouth with warm water five minutes later. Effective for cleaning teeth.

Recipe: *Gaoben san*

Rhizoma Ligustici	1 g

Ligni Aquilariae	1 g
Herba Asari	1 g
Flos Caryophylli	1 g
Gypsum Lamelliforme	30 g

Grind the above drugs into fine powder. Gargle oral cavity with warm water. Then brush teeth with a right amount of the powder. Gargle mouth with warm water five minutes later. Effective for cleaning teeth and preventing caries

Recipe: **Longhuarui san**

Ophicalcitum	60 g
Rhizoma Cimicifugae	30 g
Radix Pruni	30 g
Radix Rehmanniae	30 g
Cortex Lycii Radicis	30 g
Fructus Tribuli	30 g
Semen Armeniacae Amarum	30 g
Herba Asari	15 g
Borneolum Syntheticum	1 g
Moschus	1 g

Grind the above drugs into fine powder. Gargle oral cavity with warm water. Then brush teeth with a right amount of the powder. Gargle mouth with warm water five minutes later. Effective for cleaning teeth when the patient manifests syndrome of wind-heat stagnating in teeth. Contraindicated for pregnant women.

Recipe: **Duhuo wan**

Radix Angelicae Pubescentis	30 g
Radix Ledebouriellae	30 g
Rhizoma Ligustici Chuanxiong	30 g
Herba Asari	30 g
Radix Angelicae Sinensis	
Ligni Aquilariae	30 g
Radix Rehmanniae	30 g
Caryophylli	15 g

Melilotus Officinalis	15 g
Rhizoma Cimicifugae	15 g
Radix Glycyrrhizae	15 g

Grind the above drugs into fine powder and make it into honeyed pills. Each weighs about 1 g. Take one pill in mouth and swallow the medicated saliva. Suitable for cases manifesting *blood*-deficiency leading to malnutrition of teeth.

Chapter Fifteen
Chilblain

Chilblain is called *Dòngchuāng* in traditional Chinese medicine. When the body exposed to severe cold, some erythema and blisters will appear on certain part of the skin, especially the hand, foot, ear, nose, etc., then they will ulcerate, which is called "chilblain".

Etiology and Pathogenesis

This disorder is due to stagnation of qi and blood caused by local obstruction of the channels and collaterals. And this local obstruction is result from general debility after severe diseases, hunger, fatigue, thin cloths and too small headgears and shoes and socks in cold winter, lack of exercise and cold – resistance, and affection of exogenous cold pathogen.

Main Symptoms and Signs

Local injury seen in mild cases and common in the hand, foot, nose tip, auricle or cheeks on the pale and cold skin of which there are erythemas; burning – pain, numbness, itching, or blisters, and obvious swelling, damaged superficial or all layers of the skin, and no scar left after cure; anesthetic and analgesic affected part in severe cases, of which the skin changes from pallor successively to blue and black, around which there are swelling and big hematic blisters, on which dry or damp gangrene are even caused, infection of which may be accompanied by shiver, high fever, etc., from which if toxins sink into the interior, the patient's life is endangered, and cure of which is followed by scar.

Chapter Fifteen

Main Points of Diagnosis

1. It occurs in winter and is common among the youth and those working outdoors in winter. It usually attacks the hands, feet, face or external ears.

2. At first, the affected skin becomes pale, red and swollen and then a purplish swollen mass or a hard lump about the size of a grain of broad or maize occurs. The edge of the mass is bright red, and then the blisters and purplish blisters will appear. Some of them may have secondary infection, and even form ulceration.

3. The patient with chilblain feels itching on the affected part, has a sense of swelling, and aches when ulceration occurs.

4. The chilblain can last about one to two months and the patient will get better when the weather becomes warmer.

Differentiation and Treatment of Syndromes

1. External Treatment

1) **mild symptoms**

Local cold injury is treated in this way. The limb with cold injury is steeped in warm water of 35℃ - 40℃ as soon as possible for 5 - 7 minutes and then dried and kept warm, avoiding to be roasted from fire, rubbed with snow or soaked in cold water.

Localized burning, painful and itching, erythemas without blisters are treated with any of the following means.

(1) *Yanghe jiening gao* is applied externally.

(2) Warm decoction of such drugs as *Rhizoma Zingiberis Recens* 30 g, *Fructus Capsici* 5 ones and *Pericarpium Zanthoxyli* 10 g is used to steep and wash the affected part for 30 minutes. Then **Ointment for treating frostbite** is applied to the dried affected part. The above is done once daily.

(3) Fumigating and Washing Therapy: Take 10 grams each of *Caulis Solani*, *Caulis Capsici*, *Folium Artemisiae Argyi*, and *Cortex Cinnamomi* and decoct them in water. Use the lotion to wash the affected part, 30 minutes each time, once or twice daily.

(4) Recipe: **Tincture of Flos Carthami**

Succus Zingiberis Recens	150 ml

Chilblain

Flos Carthami	90 g
Camphorae	90 g
75% alcohol	3000 ml

Dressing change with the tincture is performed.

2) severe symptoms

The affected part is warmed and kept warm and dry. The necrotic tissue is cut off it it can be separated from the normal one. Skin grafting may be done on larger surface of wound and routine dressing change for surgical infection is conducted on smaller surface.

2. Internal Treatment

Mild cold injury, generally speaking, there is no need to take any medicine. Severe cold injury, internal therapy may be taken.

1) blood stasis due to cold

Main Symptoms and Signs: Some parts of the skin become pale or purplish with some red masses and scleromata.

Therapeutic Principles: Promoting blood circulation by warming the channels.

Recipe:

Radix Angelicae Sinensis	12 g
Radix Paeoniae Alba	12 g
Ramulus Cinnmomi	9 g
Caulis Aristolochiae Manshuriensis	6 g
Radix Glycyrrhizae Praeparata	6 g
Herba Asari	3 g
Rhizoma Zingiberis Recens	5 slices
Fructus Ziziphi Jujubae	5 fruits

Decoct the above ingredients in a right amount of water for oral administration.

Recipe:

Ramulus Cinnamomi	12 g
Radix Paeoniae Alba	12 g
Radix Angelicae Sinensis	15 g

Caulis Spatholobi	15 g
Radix Aconiti Lateralis Praeparata	10 g
Rhizoma Ligustici Chuanxiong	10 g
Radix Glycyrrhizae	10 g
Rhizoma Zingiberis Recens	10 g
Fructus Jujubae	3 dates
millet wine	30 ml

Decoct the above ingredients in a right amount of water for oral administration. Take the decoction when it is warm.

Modification: In case of general debility and deficiency of qi and blood, the drugs added are *Radix Astragali* 15 g, *Radix Rehmanniae Praeparata* 15 g, *Radix Ginseng* 10 g, *Rhizoma Atractylodis Macrocephalae* 10 g.

2) **heat transference from cold**

Main Symptoms and Signs: There are erythema, scleromata and ulceration on the affected part of the skin, accompanied with pus or scabs, and local redness and swelling.

Therapeutic Principles: Clearing away pathogenic heat and removing toxin and regulating the ying system and removing stasis.

Recipe:

Rhizoma Coptidis	9 g
Radix Scutellariae	9 g
Fructus Gardeniae	9 g
Cortex Phellodendri	9 g
Radix Angelicae Sinensis	12 g
Rhizoma Ligustici Chuanxiong	12 g
Radix Angelicae Dahuricae	12 g
Radix Paeoniae Rubra	15 g
Radix Salviae Miltiorrhizae	15 g

Decoct the above ingredients in a right amount of water for oral administration.

3) **secondary infection after ulceration**

Routine treatment of surgical infective diseases is needed and antibiotics, antitetanic serum and an tigas-gangrene serum may be considerable if necessary.

Chilblain

Prevention and Nursing

1. Do physical exercises, to strengthen the body's ability of resistance to cold. Keep the body warm and prevent coldness in winter.

2. Be sure not to rub and press the affected part, so as to protect the skin from being ulcerated and injured.

Part Two
Commonly Used Drugs

Radix Ginseng

Source The root (or with rhizome) of *Panax ginseng* C.A. Mey., family *Araliaceae*.

Characteristics 1. Dried wild ginseng: Axial root short and broad, often bifurcate, 2 – 10 cm long, grayish yellow – white; cork lenticellate and longitudinally striped, with annular marks at the upper part. Fibrous root numerous, slender, with granular protuberances. Rhizome slender, somewhat curved, cambium visible. Hard in texture.

2. Dried cultivated ginseng: Axial root about 15 cm long, 1 – 2 cm in diameter, with 2 – 3 branches and few fibrous roots, sometimes with granular protuberances, and slender adventitious roots.

3. Steamed and dried cultivated ginseng: Axial root terete, 10 cm long, remained with 2 – 3 branches, translucent, reddish brown. Section even, flat and corneous. All are sweet and slightly bitter in taste, warm in nature, and attributive to spleen, lung and heart meridians.

Indication 1. Invigorate vital energy and relieve collapse – syndrome: For collapse – syndrome with listlessness, weak respiration and indistinct pulse; single use for exhaustion of vital energy or blood (Decoction of *Ginseng*); for *yin* – exhaustion, used together with **Radix Ophiopogonis**, **Fructus Schisandrae** (Powder for Restoring Pulse); for *yang* – exhaustion, used together with **Radix Aconiti Praeparata** (Decoction of *Radix Ginseng* and *Radix Aconiti Praeparata*).

2. Invigorate spleen – energy: For spleen – deficiency syndrome manifest-

ed by poor appetite, fatigue and emaciation, hemorrhagic diseases, prolapse of uterus and rectum, visceroptosis and anemia.

3. Promote the production of body fluid to quench thirst: For febrile diseases with consumption of body fluid, and diabetes.

4. Invigorate lung - energy: for deficiency of lung - energy manifested by shortness of breath, dyspnea, cough, night sweat, and susceptibility to common cold.

5. Invigorate *wei* - energy: For common cold in debilitated patient, pyogenic skin infection and carbuncle of *yin* type.

6. Supplement vital energy and calm the mind: For deficiency of heart energy manifested by palpitation, amnesia, insomnia, absent - mindedness, spontaneous perspiration, cardiodynia, etc.. In addition, also for impotence, sterility, emission, ejaculatio praecox, enuresis, etc..

Selected Recipes 1. For hoariness:

Radix Ginseng	150 g
dried *Radix Rehmanniae Praeparata*	300 g
Radix Asparagi	300 g
Poria	300 g
shelled *Semen Cannabis*	300 g

Pound and grind the above drugs into fine powder. Make the powder into pills with honey, each weighs about 3 g. Take 10 pills after breakfast with warm millet wine.

2. For acne:

Recipe: *Wu shen san*

Radix Ginseng	3 g
Radix Salviae Miltiorrhizae	3 g
Radix Sophorae Flavescentis	30 g
Radix Glehniae	30 g
Radix Scutellariae	30 g
Semen Juglandis	15 g

Grind the first five drugs into fine powder. Pound *Semen Juglandis* into mash. Make the powder into pills with the mash. Each weighs about 3 g. Take 30 pills with tea after meals, three times daily.

3. For looseness of teeth and hoariness by dispersing wind and regulating

qi:

Recipe: Miao ying san

Radix Ginseng	15 g
Rhizoma Cyperi	15 g
Herba Asari	15 g
Poria	15 g
Rhizoma Ligustici Chuanxiong	15 g
Fructus Tribuli	15 g
Fructus Amomi	15 g
Radix Angelicae Dahuricae	20 g
Gypsum Fibrosum	20 g
Os Draconis	20 g
Moschus	a small amount

Grind the above drugs into fine powder. Gargle the mouth with a cup of warm water with a right amount of powder, twice daily.

4. For facial hemiparalysis due to apoplexy:

Recipe: Ren shen wan

Radix Ginseng	30 g
Radix Aconiti	30 g
Rhizoma Achyranthis Bidentatae	30 g

Grind them into powder and make pills with paste of wheat flour, each weighs about 1 g. Take 10 pills with millet, twice daily.

Modern Research *Radix Ginseng* and *Radix Glycyrrhizae* 20 g each, *Radix Astragali seu Hedysari* 50 g, *Radix Paeoniae Alba* and *Cortex Cinnamomi* 30 g each, *Rhizoma Atractylodis Macrocephalae*, *Radix Rehmanniae Praeparata* and *Radix Polygoni Multiflori* 45 g each, *Fructus Ziziphi Jujubae* 20 g, *Mel* 500 g are ground into fine powder except *Mel*. Make the powder into pills with honey. Each pill weighs 10 g and contains 10 g of raw drugs. Take the one pill each time, three times daily. It is effective for calvities. *Fructus Schisandrae*, *Radix Polygalae* and *Semen Biotae* are added for dizziness, insomnia and amnesia; *Fructus Lycii*, *Semen Cuscutae* and *Fructus Psoraleae* added for lumbago and soreness of the lower extremities.

Radix et Rhizoma Rhei

Source The root and rhizome of *Rheum palmatum* L, *R. tanguticum* Maxim. ex Balf. or *R. officinale* Baill., family *Polygonaceae*.

Characteristics Crude drug nearly terete, conical or lecotropal, 5 - 15 cm long, 2 - 8 cm in diameter; surface yellow - brown, sometimes with residual cork. Prepared as transversely cut pieces. The section of rhizome showing narrow cortex and wood, broad pith with alternating yellow - brown and red - brown striae and numerous peculia vascular bundles in asteriate annular arrangement or scattered; the section of the root showing developed xylem, radially arranged vascular bundles and visible annular marks. Delicately aromatic in odor. Bitter in taste, cold in nature, and attributive to spleen, stomach, large intestine, liver and pericardium meridians.

Indication 1. Promote digestion and relieve dyspepsia, purge heat and clear away toxic materials: (1) for constipation of sthenia - heat type with coma, delirium, convulsion, mania or abdominal distention and pain, usually used together with *Natrii Sulphas*, *Fructus Aurantii Immaturus*, *Cortex Magnoliae Officinalis*, (Decoction for Potent Purgation); (2) for syndrome resulting from evils accumulating in the thorax with abdominal distention and pain, tenderness, dry tongue and thirst, hectic fever, or shortness of breath and restlessness, used together with *Radix Euphorbiae Kansui*, *Natrii Sulphas* (Decoction for Severe Phlegm - Heat Syndrome in the Chest); (3) for acute appendicitis, usually used together with *Cortex Moutan Radicis*, *Semen Persicae*; (4) for dysentery of dampness - heat type with abdominal pain and tenesmus, used together with *Fructus Aurantii Immaturus*, *Rhizoma Coptidis*, etc.; (5) for acute and simple intestinal obstruction, roundworm intestinal obstruction and paralytic intestinal obstruction, Decoction for Potent Purgation may be used; (7) for food and dug poisoning; (8) for pulmonary heart disease with respiratory failure and constipation; (9) for uremia, decoction as enema may be used; (10) for cold - syndrome with constipation, used together with *Radix Aconiti Praeparata*, *Rhizoma Zingiberis Recens*, etc..

2. Clear away heat and toxic materials: Oral and external use for furuncle and carbuncle due to intense heat; topical use for burn of medium or small size, cervical erosion and mycotic vaginitis; for furunculosis complicated by sep-

ticemia, used together with *Flos. Lonicerae*, *Fructus Forsythiae*, *etc.*; also for sore throat, conjunctival conestion, aphthae and toothache due to domination of fire.

3. Stop bleeding: For peptic ulcer with bleeding, also for hemoptysis and epistaxis due to blood stasis, blood − heat or domination of fire; external use for traumatic bleeding.

4. Promote blood circulation and remove blood stasis: For trauma, especially those of the chest and abdomen with constipation; anemia, dysmenorrhea and postpartum abdominal pain due to blood stasis.

5. Chologogue and relieve jaundice: For preventing and treating icterus neonatorum (including ABO type hemolytic jaundice of newborn), used together with *Herba Artemisiae Scopariae*, *Radix Scutellariae*, *Radix Glycyrrhizae*; for icteric viral jaundice, and acute and serious cases of hepatitis.

Administration 3 − 12 g. Powder: 2 − 5 g, daily dose 4 − 10 g. For purgation, decoct later (only boil for less than 10 minutes) or soak in the boiled water for oral use.

Selected Recipes For acne: Powder of *Radix et Rhizoma Rhei*. Mix the powder with water and apply it on the affected part after supper, once daily.

For alopecia areata: Grind equal dose of *Radix et Rhizoma Rhei* and *Radix Scutellariae* into fine powder. Mix the powder with a right amount of millet wine and apply the mixture on the affected part.

For brandy nose: Grind equal dose of *Radix et Rhizoma Rhei*, *Natrii Sulphas* and *Semen Arecae* into fine powder and apply the powder on the affected part. Change the powder once daily. Clean up the affected part three days later. Pound raw ginkgo into mash and apply it on the affected part.

Grind Grind equal dose of *Radix et Rhizoma Rhei* and *Sulfur* into fine powder. Mix the powder with a right amount of water and apply the mixture on the affected part. Effective for acne rosacea.

For toothache, gingival bleeding and halitosis: Grind carbonized *Radix et Rhizoma Rhei* into fine powder. Brush the teetch with the powder.

For chilblain: Grind *Radix et Rhizoma Rhei* into fine powder. Apply the powder on the affected part.

Caution Contraindicated for those with superficial syndrome, deficiency of both *qi* and *blood*, asthenic coldness in the spleen and stomach due to deficiency of *yang*; cases without sthenic heat, stagnation or blood stasis. Pregnant women prohibited.

Modern Research For seborrheic dermatitis: 100 g of *Radix et Rhizoma Rhei* and 20 g of *Borneolum Syntheticum* are soaked in 250 g of edible vinegar in a sealed jar for seven days. Filter the leachate for later use. Disinfect the affect part with 75% alcohol, the apply a right amount of the leachate on the affected part, three to four times daily. Some severe cases were given treatment of clearing away internal heat. 45 cases with seborrheic dermatitis were treated with the above therapy. Among them, 20 cases recovered completely, 15 cases improved considerably, 5 cases received some effect and the other 5 cases failed to received any effect.

Rhizoma Dioscoreae

Source Rhizome of *Dioscorea opposita* Thunb., family *Dioscoreaceae*.

Characteristics Rhizome terete or long cambiform, somewhat curved, 15 – 30 cm long, 1.5 – 6.0 cm in diameter. Surface with yellowish white cork, and appearing white when the cork is peeled off. Prepared as oblique cutting pieces, white, farinaceous, even, and without striae. Sweet in taste, mild in nature, and attributive to spleen, lung and kidney meridians.

Indication 1. Invigorate the spleen and stomach: For deficiency of spleen energy and stomach – energy with poor appetite, fatigue, loose stools or chronic diarrhea, leukorrhagia, etc.; for febrile diseases with consumption of body fluid or deficiency of spleen – *yin* and stomach – *yin* with poor appetite, thirst, dry tongue, diabetes, etc..

    2. Invigorate the lung: For lung – deficiency with chronic cough or tuberculosis; for deficiency of lung and kidney with dyspnea and chronic cough, used together with *Fructus Corni* and *Fructus Schisandrae*.

    3. Invigorate the kidney and preserve the essence: For kidney – deficiency manifested as emission, enuresis, frequent micturition and leukorrhagia.

Administration Decoction: 10 – 30 g.

Selected Recipes For invigorating the deficiency and improving complexion:

Recipe: *Shuyu wan*

Rhizoma Dioscoreae	30 g
Herba Cistanchis	30 g
Radix Rehmanniae Praeparata	30 g
Semen Cuscutae	30 g
Radix Aconiti Praeparata	30 g
lapis rubrum	30 g
Rhizoma Achyranthis Bidentatae	30 g
Fructus Schisandrae	30 g
Rhizoma Alismatis	30 g
Fructus Corni	30 g
Poria	30 g
Radix Morindae Officinalis	30 g
Semen Biotae	30 g
Cortex Cinnamomi	30 g
Radix Ginseng	30 g
Rhizoma Atractylodis Macrocephalae	30 g
Rhizoma Zingiberis	30 g

Grind the above drugs into fine powder and make the powder pills with honey. Each pill weighs about 6 g. Take 10 pills before breakfast with warm water.

For regulating ying and wei, relieving pain in the extremities and dispersing wind-cold:

Recipe: *Shengji shuyu wan*

Rhizoma Dioscoreae	30 g
Fructus Rubi	30 g
Radix Rehmanniae Praeparata	60 g
Fructus Schisandrae	30 g
Rhizoma Dioscoreae Bishie	30 g
Fructus Cnidii	30 g
Herba Cistanchis	30 g
Radix Polygalae	30 g
Semen Cuscutae	60 g
Herba Dendrobii	30 g

Cortex Cinnamomi	45 g
Cortex Eucommiae	45 g
Fructus Corni	30 g
Radix Ginseng	30 g
Radix Ledebouriellae	30 g
Cortex Acanthopanacis Radicis	9 g
Rhizoma Cibotii	30 g
Radix Astragali seu Hedysari	30 g
Radix Gentianae Macrophyllae	30 g
Rhizoma Atractylodis Macrocephalae	30 g
Radix Ophiopogonis	45 g
Radix Morindae Officinalis	30 g

Grind the above drugs into fine powder and make the powder pills with honey. Each pill weighs about 3 g. Take 30 pills before breakfast with warm millet wine.

Modern Research For moth-patch: 20 g of *Rhizoma Dioscoreae*, 18 g of *Radix Rehmanniae Praeparata*, 15 g of *Poria* and *Rhizoma Alismatis* each, 12 g of *Flos Chrysanthemi* and *Cortex Phellodendri* each, 9 g of *Cortex Moutan Radicis*, *Fructus Corni*, *Fructus Lycii* and *Pericarpium Citri Reticulatae* each. The recipe consisting of the above drugs was used for cases with moth-patch. In cases of blood insufficiency, 15 g of *Radix Polygoni Multiflori* added; add 20 g of *Caulis Spatholobi* and 12 g of *Flos Carthami* for blood stasis; in cases of insomnia, 30 g of *Caulis Polygoni Multiflori* and 15 g of *Cortex Albiziae* added. 98 cases with moth-patch were given the treatment. Among them, 46 recovered completely, 31 cases improved considerably, 18 cases received effect of some degree, 3 cases failed to receive any effect after taking 6-32 doses.

Fructus Corni

Source The pulp of *Cornus officinalis* Sieb. et Zucc., family *Cornaceae*.
Characteristics Pulp appearing as irregular sacs or flat pieces, about 1 cm in size, purple-red to purple-black wrinkled, lustrous; tip with residual persis-

tent calyx, base with residual fruit stalk. Soft in texture. Sour and astringent in taste, slightly warm in nature, and attributive to liver and kidney meridians.

Indication   1. Invigorate the liver and kidney, supplement the essence and improve visual acuity. For deficiency of the liver and kidney manifested by soreness of the waist and knees, flaccidity of the lower limbs, impotence, frequent micturition, sterility, dizziness, tinnitus and blurring of vision.

2. Astringe and preserve essence: For hypofunction of liver and kidney manifested by emission, enuresis, frequency of micturition, metrorrhagia, menorrhagia, spontaneous perspiration, night sweat, collpase with profuse perspiration and dyspnea of asthenic type.

Administration   Decoction: 6 – 12 g, up to 30 g.

Selected Recipes   For dim complexion due to deficiency of kidney – *yang*:

Recipe: *Ba wei wan*

Cortex Moutan Radicis	90 g
Poria	90 g
Rhizoma Alismatis	90 g
Radix Rehmanniae Praeparata	240 g
Fructus Corni	120 g
Rhizoma Dioscoreae	120 g
Radix Aconiti Praeparata	60 g
Cortex Cinnamomi	120 g

The above drugs are ground into fine powder. Make the powder with a right amount of *Mel* into pills, each weighs about 1 g. Take 15 to 25 pills with warm millet wine on an empty stomach, twice daily.

For regulating ying and wei in order to improving the complexion:

Recipe: *Lingyangzi muxiang wan*

Fructus Corni	30 g
Poria	60 g
Radix Aucklandiae	60 g
Flos Nelumbinis	30 g
Fructus Psoraleae	150 g
Semen Cuscutae	150 g
Semen Juglandis	240 g

The above drugs are ground into fine powder. Make the powder with a right amount of *Mel* into pills, each weighs about 1 g. Take seventy pills with warm millet wine on an empty stomach, once daily.

Rhizoma Ligustici Chuanxiong

Source The rhizome of *Ligusticum chuanxiong* Hort., family *Umbelliferae*.

Characteristics Rhizome nodular fist − like masses, 1.5 − 7.0 cm in diameter. Surface yellow − brown, with many dense stem nodes, protruding, with rounded depressed stem scars on the upper part, and many tubercular root scars on the lower pat and nodes. Prepared as crosscutting pieces, margin of the pieces irregularly wavy, grey − yellow. Annular wavy cambium, and brown oily spots scattered. Strongly aromatic in odor. Acrid and bitter in taste, warm in nature, and attributive to liver, gallbladder and pericardium meridians.

Indication 1. Promote the circulation of blood and vital energy: For stagnation of blood and vital energy resulting in angina pectoris, headache, chest pain, abdominal pain, dysmenorrhea, amenorrhea, difficult menstruation, dead fetus and retention of placenta, apoplexy, traumata, bony spur, or thromboangiitis obliterans.

2. Expel wind and alleviate pain: For recurrent headache, dizziness, headache of wind − cold type and rheumatism. Also sued for leukocytopenia.

Administration Decoction: 3 − 9 g; 9 − 15 g for severe cases.

Selected Recipes For halitosis:

Recipe: From *Qianjin fang*

Rhizoma Ligustici Chuanxiong	120 g
Radix Angelicae Dahuricae	120 g
Pericarpium Citri Reticulatae	120 g
Cortex Cinnamomi	120 g
Fructus Ziziphi Jujubae with stones removed	240 g

Grind the drugs except *Fructus Ziziphi Jujubae* into fine powder. Mix the powder with *Fructus Ziziphi Jujubae*. Make the mixture into pills with size similar to a soybean! Take 10 pills around mealtime. One course consists of seven continuous days of treatment.

For foul breath due to caries:

Recipe 1

Rhizoma Ligustici Chuanxiong	30 g
Radix Angelicae Dahuricae	30 g
Radix Glycyrrhizae	9 g
Cortex Cinnamomi	15 g
wildginger	15 g
Radix Angelicae Sinensis	9 g

Grind the drugs into fine powder. Take 3 g with warm millet wine on an empty stomach, twice daily. One course consists of thirty continuous days of treatment.

Recipe 2

Rhizoma Ligustici Chuanxiong	30 g
Radix Angelicae Sinensis	30 g
Radix Angelicae Pubescentis	30 g
Herba Asari	30 g
Radix Angelicae Dahuricae	30 g

Pound the drugs into powder. Decoct 15 g of the powder in a right amount of water. Filter the decoction to make gargle. Gargle the mouth when it is warm.

For odontoseisis and toothache:

Recipe 1: *Xiongqiong tang*

Rhizoma Ligustici Chuanxiong	45 g
Radix Ledebouriellae	30 g
Semen Coicis	30 g
Herba Asari	15 g

Pound the drugs into powder. Decoct 5 g of the powder in a right amount of water. Filter the decoction to make gargle. Gargle the mouth when it is warm.

Recipe 2

Rhizoma Ligustici Chuanxiong	60 g
Herba Asari	30 g
Radix Ledebouriellae	30 g

Commonly Used Drugs

Semen Coicis	60 g
Cortex Lycii Radicis	30 g
Cacumen Tamaricis	30 g

Pound the drugs into powder. Decoct 15 g of the powder in a right amount of water. Filter the decoction to make gargle. Gargle the mouth when it is warm.

For acne:

Recipe: Yangshi jiacang tang

Rhizoma Ligustici Chuanxiong	30 g
Rhizoma seu Radix Notopterygii	30 g
Radix Ledebouriellae	30 g
Flos Chrysanthemi	30 g
Fructus Tribuli	30 g
Radix Glycyrrhizae	30 g
Fructus Gardeniae	9 g

Grind the above drugs into fine powder. Take 6 g orally with tea after meals.

Recipe: Meishi qingfei tang

Rhizoma Ligustici Chuanxiong
Fructus Forsythiae
Radix Angelicae Dahuricae
Rhizoma Coptidis
Radix Scutellariae
Herba Schizonepetae
Ramulus Mori
Fructus Gardeniae
Bulbus Fritillariae Cirrhosae
Radix Glycyrrhizae

All the above drugs are to be decocted in water for oral administration.

For odontoseisis and grey hair:

Recipe 1

Rhizoma Ligustici Chuanxiong	60 g
Herba Asari	60 g
Herba Schizonepetae	60 g

Radix Angelicae Sinensis	60 g
edible salt	120 g

Pound and grind the above drugs into fine powder and heat the powder over fire. Store the carbonized powder for later use. Apply a right amount of powder on teeth, twice daily.

Recipe 2

Rhizoma Ligustici Chuanxiong	30 g
Herba Ecliptae	60 g
Radix Angelicae Sinensis	30 g
Fructus Gleditsiae	15 g
Radix Angelicae Dahuricae	15 g
Poria	30 g
edible salt	75 g
Cortex Phellodendri	15 g

Grind the above drugs into fine powder and store the powder in a sealed jar. Heat the jar over until the powder has been carbonized. Apply a right amount of powder on teeth before breakfast and rub the gingivae to and fro for times.

Caution Contraindicated for cases with hyperactivity of fire-heat due to deficiency of kidney-yin, or cases with deficiency of qi.

Modern Research 3 ml of 10% Injectio Rhizoma Ligustici Chuanxiong and 3 ml of 10% Injectio Radix Ledebouriellae is mixed. Inject the mixed injection on both sides of **Xuèhǎi**(SP10) and **Fēngchí**(GB20). Each point is injected 1.5 ml, once daily or once other day. 14 cases with flat wart were given the above treatment. Among them, 6 cases fully recovered, 5 cases received considerable effect, 2 cases improved in some degree, while one case failed to receive any effect. One to two years of follow-ups revealed satisfactory effects on 6 cases who recovered completely.

Fructus Ligustri Lucidi

Source Fruit of *Ligustrum lucidum* Ait., family *Oleaceae*.

Characteristics Fruit elliptical or reniform, 6.0-8.5 mm long, 3.5-5.5 mm in diameter. Surface purple - dark, irregularly wrinkled. Pericarp thin, easily to be separated; pulp loose and soft; kernel yellow - brown, with longitudinal ridges, containing one seed. Sweet and bitter in taste, slightly cld in nature, and attributive to liver and kidney meridians.

Indication　1. Tonify the liver and the kidney, darken the hair and promote the visual acuity: For deficiency of liver - *yin* and kidney - *yin* manifested as dizziness, tinnitus, blurring of vision, weakness of the loin and knees, hectic fever, nocturnal emission, alopecia and poliosis, usually used with *Herba Ecliptae* (*Erzhi* Pill). Recently also used for seborrheic alopecia, central retinitis, early cataract, etc..

2. Tranquilize the mind by nourishing the heart: For insufficiency of heart - *yin* manifested as insomnia, palpitation and precordial pain. Recently, also used for angina pectoris, hyperlipemia and neurasthenia, especially those of *yin* - deficiency type. In addition, also used for leukocytopenia, viral hepatitis with *yin* - deficiency syndrome; its component oleanolic acid for various kinds of hepatitis.

Administration　Decoction: 9 - 15 g.

Selected Recipes　For grey hair due to deficiency of kidney - *yin*:

　　Recipe: *Erzhi wan*

　　　Fructus Ligustri Lucidi

　　　Herba Ecliptae

Grind dried shelled *Fructus Ligustri Lucidi* into powder. Pound *Herba Ecliptae* and extract the juice. Mix the powder with the juice and make pills with the mixture. Take the pills at bedtime.

Caution　Contraindicated for cases with deficiency of spleen - *yang* and stomach - *yang*.

Radix Polygoni Multiflori

Source　Root tuber of *Polygonum multiflorum* Thunb., family *Polygonaceae*. That prepared by drying is known as crude sample, and that prepared by steaming with the juice of black soya beans as prepared sample.

Characteristics　Crude sample: Root tuber irregularly cambiform, 6 - 15 cm long, 4 – 12 cm in diameter. Cork red – brown, wrinkled, with transverse and long lenticels and spotted fibrous root scars. Prepared by crosscutting, the section appearing reddish brown; the cortex with several special vascular bundles in annular arrangement like cloudy striae, the middle being vascular bundles of the xylem, somewhat rounded. hard in texture, heavy in weight. Prepared sample: which is similar to the former except it is dark – brown in color and the cloudy stria indistinct. Both of them are bitter, astringent and sweet in taste, warm in nature, and attributive to liver, heart and kidney meridians.

Indication 1. Invigorate the liver and kidney, benefit essence and blood: For insufficiency of essence and blood manifested as baldness, backache with weakness of the knee joint, immovability of the extremities, hemiplegia and paraplegia; for blood – deficiency syndrome manifested as sallow complexion, palpitation, dizziness, tinnitus, numbness of the extremities, insomnia, dreaminess sleepiness, somnambulism, epilepsy, urticaria and dermatoxerasia; for hypofunction of liver and kidney with emission or leukorrhagia. Recently, also used for hypercholesterinemia and atherosclerosis.

2. Relax the bowels (crude herb): For constipation of asthenia – syndrome.

3. Clear away toxic maerial (crude herb): For scrofula, carbuncle, etc.. In addition, the prepared herb is used for chronic malaria with deficiency of vital energy and blood.

Administration Decoction: 9 – 25 g.

Selected Recipes For Invigorating kidney – essence and darkening grey hair:

Recipe: *Puji heshouwu wan*

Radix Polygoni Multiflori	240 g
Herba Cistanchis	180 g
Rhizoma Achyranthis Bidentatae	120 g

Steam the drugs with a right amount of Chinese dates for half an hour. Then dry the drugs in the sun. Grind the dried drugs into powder and make pills with it. Each pills weighs about 1 g. Take 5 to 7 pills with warm millet wine, three times daily. Take extra one pill prior to meals.

Recipe: *Qibao meiran dan*

Radix Polygoni Multiflori	1000 g
Poria	1000 g

Rhizoma Achyranthis Bidentatae	240 g
Radix Angelicae Sinensis	240 g
Fructus Lycii	240 g
Semen Cuscutae	240 g
Fructus Psoraleae	120 g

Grind the dried drugs into powder and make it into honeyed pills. Among them, 150 pills weigh about 6 g each, others about 0.2 g each. Take one big pill with warm millet wine in the morning, one with ginger soup at noon and one with salt water at bedtime. Take other 100 small pills on an empty stomach, once daily.

For odontoseisis and grey hair by invigorating kidney essence:

Recipe: *Jifeng sizhu wan*

Radix Polygoni Multiflori	120 g
Rhizoma Acori Graminei	120 g
Rhizoma Achyranthis Bidentatae	120 g
Radix Aconiti	120 g

Pound the above drugs except **Radix Aconiti** into powder and steam it with 3 liters of millet wine until it is dried. Grind **Radix Aconiti** into powder and mix it with the prepared powder of the other three drugs. Make pills with the mixed powder. Take 20 g on an empty stomach, once daily.

For darkening grey hair and improving complexion:

Recipe: *Shengji shouwu wan*

Radix Polygoni Multiflori	720 g
Rhizoma Acori Calami	240 g
Rhizoma Achyranthis Bidentatae	480 g
Rhizoma Arisaematis	120 g

Grind the dried drugs into powder and mix it with 5 liters of vinegar and 10 liters of millet wine. Heat the mixture in an earthenware pot until the mixture becomes some kind of extract. Make pills with the extract, each weighs about 2 g. Take 10 pills with warm salt water on an empty stomach.

For sleeking skin and strengthening muscles:

Recipe: *Heshouwu wan*

Radix Polygoni Multiflori	480 g
Radix Paeoniae Rubra	120 g

      Rhizoma Achyranthis Bidentatae   120 g

      Radix Rehmanniae Praeparata   120 g

    Grind the above drugs into fine powder and make pills, each weighs about 1 g. Take 30 pills with warm millet wine on an empty stomach.

Modern Research   Shouwu jinyingzi tang (*prepared Radix Polygoni Multiflori* 15 – 45 g, *Fructus Rosae Laevigatae* 30 g, *Fructus Lycii*, *Radix Angelicae Sinensis*, *Rhizoma Polygonati*, *Radix Astragali seu Hedysari*, *Rhizoma Atractylodis Macrocephalae*, *Radix Rehmanniae Praeparata*, *gordon euryale*, *Semen Biotae* 15 each), one dose daily; prepared *Radix Polygoni Multiflori* and *Fructus Rosae Laevigatae* 60 g each soaked in spirits for one week. Apply the filtered tincture on the affected part, three times daily. 14 cases with pelade were given the above treatment. All recovered within 20 to 45 days. **Shouwu tang** (*Radix Polygoni Multiflori*, *Radix Rehmanniae Praeparata*, *Fructus Lycii*, *Fructus Ligustri Lucidi* 15 g each, *Rhizoma Cimicifugae* 5 g, *Radix Polygalae* 6 g, *Semen Cuscutae*, *Semen Biotae* 9 g each, *Herba Ecliptae* 12 g, *Poria*, *Radix Angelicae Sinensis*, *Colla Corii Asini* 10 g each), one dose daily for 10 to 20 days; Rub the affected part one slice of ginger for one to two minutes, twice daily. 10 cases with pelade recovered completely after taking 7 to 20 doses. *Radix Polygoni Multiflori*, *Semen Phaseoli* 20 g each, *Semen Cannabis*, *Radix Astragali seu Hedysari*, *Colla Corii Asini* 15 g each, *Rhizoma Atractylodis Macrocephalae*, *Arillus Longan* 12 g each, *Fructus Ziziphi Jujubae* 19 dates, one dose daily, one course consisting of 20 doses; Apply decoction of *Cortex Mori Radicis* on the affected part, twice to three times daily. 50 cases recovered after one to three courses of treatment. Follow – ups within 3 – 5 years revealed no recurrence.

    Prepared *Radix Polygoni Multiflori* and *Radix Rehmanniae Praeparata* 30 g each, and 15 g of *Radix Angelicae Sinensis* soaked in 1000 ml of white spirits and sealed for 10 – 15 days. Take 15 – 30 ml daily. 36 cases with grey hair were given the above treatment. Among them, 24 cases fully recovered (20 circumscribed cases and 4 diffuse cases), 8 cases improved, 4 cases got no response.

    20 g of *Radix Polygoni Multiflori*, 10 g of *sappan wood*, *Fructus Leonuri*, *Periostracum Cicadae*, *Radix Paeoniae Rubra* each, 15 g of *Fructus Tribuli*, 6 dates of *Fructus Ziziphi Jujubae*. Add *Radix Rehman-*

niae, *Radix Rehmanniae Praeparata*, *Fructus Lycii*, *Rhizoma Polygonati*, *Semen Sesami* for deficiency of liver – *yin* and kidney – *yin*; *Radix Salviae Miltiorrhizae* for blood stasis; *Poria*, *Semen Coicis*, *Radix Scutellariae* for dampness – heat. All the above drugs decocted in water for oral administration, one dose daily, one course of treatment consisting of 10 doses. Heliotherapy on the affected skin also adopted (strong insolation prohibited). 36 cases with leukoderma were given the above treatment. Among them, 20 cases recovered completely, 12 cases improved, 4 cases failed. Most cases improved within 6 to 10 months.

Radix Asparagi

Source   The root tuber of *Asparagus cochinchinensis* (Lour.) Merr., family Liliaceae.

Characteristics   Root tuber long – cambiform, slightly curved, 5 – 18 cm long. Surface withbark removed appearing yellow – white to yellow – brown, semiopaque, slightly longitudinally wrinkled. Fracture suface showing a narrow stele and a broad cortex. Soft and sticky in texture. Sweet and bitter in taste, cold in nature, and attributive to lung and kidney meridians.

Indication   Nourish *yin*, clear away heat, moisturize the lung and benefit the kidney: For *yin* – deficiency with lung – dryness manifested as dry cough, hemoptysis, dry throat and thirst; diabetes with consumption of body fluid; *yin* – deficiency with hectic fever, night sweat, nocturnal emission, flaccidity of lower limbs; constipation due to dryness of intestine.

Administration   Decoction: 5 – 15 g.

Selected Recipes   For darkening grey hair:

   Recipe: *Shenghui wufa wan*

Radix Asparagi	1000 g
Radix Rehmanniae Praeparata	480 g

Grind the above drugs into fine powder and make it with a right amount of honey into pills. Each pills weighs 1 g. Take 30 pills on an empty stomach.

   For improving complexion: Take 9 g of *Radix Asparagi* with millet wine, 5 times daily.

Caution Contraindicated for cases with deficiency of spleen − *yang* and wind − cold syndrome.

Radix Salviae Miltiorrhizae

Source The root and rhizome of *Salvia miltiorrhiza* Bunge, family *Labiatae*.

Characteristics Rhizome appearing as irregular masses with several hairy roots growing at the lower part. Root 20 − 30 cm long and 0.5 − 1.0 cm in diameter; surface red, often presenting scaly exfoliation. Prepared as segments, the section showing several rectangular vascular bundles in radial arrangement. Bitter in taste, slightly cold in nature, and attributive to heart, pericardium and liver meridians.

Indication 1. Promote blood circulation to remove blood stasis: For cardiodynia, hypochondriac pain, abdominal pain, stomachache, dysmenorrhea, amenorrhea, lochiorrhea and traumata with blood stasis, used together with *Radix Angelicae Sinensis* and *Olibani*. Recently also used for ischemic apoplexy, disseminated intravascular coagulation, chronic hepatitis, cirrhosis, etc..

2. Clear away heat, relieve vexation, nourish blood and tranquilize the mind: For seasonal febrile diseases involving yingfen and xuefen manifested by high fever, irritability, delirium and skin eruptions, usually used together with *Cornu Rhinocerotis*, *Radix Scrophulariae* and *Rhizoma Coptidis*; for insanity attributive to blood stasis and heat, used together with *Lumbricus*; also for restlessness, frightening and insomnia due to heart − heat or insufficiency of heart − *blood*.

3. Cool the *blood* to relieve carbuncle: For carbuncles and pharyngitis.

Administration Decoction: 6 − 15 g.

Selected Recipes For brandy nose:

  Recipe: *Yi bian jiuci fang*
   Radix Salviae Miltiorrhizae
   Radix Rehmanniae
   Radix Angelicae Sinensis
   Flos Carthami
   Fructus Gardeniae

Commonly Used Drugs

  Cortex Mori Radicis
  Radix Ledebouriellae
  Herba Menthae

All the above drugs are to be decocted in water for oral administration.

For acne:

Recipe: *Puji wushen wan*

Radix Ginseng	3 g
Radix Salviae Miltiorrhizae	3 g
Radix Sophorae Flavescentis	30 g
Radix Glehniae	30 g
Radix Scutellariae	30 g
Semen Juglandis	15 g

  Grind the above drugs except *Semen Juglandis* into fine powder. Pound *Semen Juglandis* along with the powder and make pills. Each weighs about 1 g. Take 30 pills after meals, three times daily.

Modern Research Tanshinone tablet (0.25 g/tab), 3 to 5 tab., t.i.d.. 23 cases with acne (16 cases with acne rosacea, 7 with acne cystica) were given the above treatment. Among them, 8 fully recovered, 13 got considerable effect, 2 improves in some degree. 20 cases with acne vulgaris, 18 cases with acne pustulosa and 8 cases with acne cystia were given the above treatment, who got considerable improvement. 15 g of *Radix Salviae Miltiorrhizae*, 12 g of *Cortex Mori Radicis*, *Radix Scutellariae*, *Fructus Gardeniae*, *Cortex Moutan Radicis* and *Radix Paeoniae Rubra* each, 9 g of *Fructus Forsythiae*, 3 g of *Radix Glycyrrhizae*, 6 g of *Radix et Rhizoma Rhei*, decocted in water for oral administration, one dose daily. 55 cases with acne were given the above treatment. Among them, 52 fully recovered and 3 failed due to stopped administration.

  60 g of *Radix Salviae Miltiorrhizae*, 15 g of *Radix Angelicae Sinensis*, 9 g of *Semen Persicae*, *Flos Carthami*, *Herba Lycopi*, *Radix Curcumae* and *Rhizoma Sparganii* each, 30 g of *Herba Leonuri* and *Radix Ilicis Pubescentis* each. Add *Rhizoma Cyperi*, *Pericarpium Citri Reticulatae* and *Pericarpium Citri Reticulatae Viride* for distending pain in the hypochondriac region. Add prepared *Radix et Rhizoma Rhei* and *Radix Scutellariae* for constipation. Add *Radix Astragali seu Hedysari* for listlessness, decocted in

water for oral administration, one dose daily. 1.5 g of powder of *Scolopendra*, three times daily. 9 cases with moth-patches were given the above treatment. Among them, 7 fully recovered after the treatment of 3 months, and 2 recovered 5 months later. Follow-ups of one year revealed no recurrence.

Radix Astragali seu Hedysari

Source Root of *Astragalus membranaceus* (Fisch.) Bunge var. *mongholicus* (Bunge) Hsiao, and *A. membranaceus* (Fisch.) Bunge, and the other species of the same genus and *Hedysarum polybotrys* Hand.-Mazz., family *Leguminosae*.

Characteristics 1. *Astragali*: Root long-terete, occasionally branching, 30 - 90 cm long, 1.0 - 3.5 cm in diameter. Cork grey-yellow, with lenticels and fibrous root scar, old root base bearing stem base, its pith often withered and dark-brown. Fracture surface fibrous and farinaceous; cortex slightly loose, fibrous and reticular. Prepared as cross or obliquely cutting pieces, section light yellow, the cortex usually separated from the xylem, vascular bundles in the xylem fine, dense and radially arranged, with cracks sometimes. Slightly sweet when chewed, with a smell of beans.

2. *Hedysari*: Cork red-brown, usually peeling off to reveal a yellow cortex. Cross section dense, cortex with sparse fibers. Both are sweet in taste, slightly warm in nature, and attributive to spleen and lung meridians.

Indication 1. Invigorate vital energy and spleen: For spleen-deficiency with poor appetite, loose stools, fatigue and bleeding, usually used together with *Radix Codonopsis Pilosulae* and *Rhizoma Atractylodis Macrocephalae*; for deficiency of both vital energy and *blood*, used together with *Radix Angelicae Sinensis* (Decoction of *Radix Angelicae Sinensis* for Enriching Blood).

2. Invigorate vital energy to activate *yang*: For collapse of middle-*jiao* manifested by prolapse of rectum, hysteroptosis or gastroptosis, usually used together with *Radix Codonopsis Pilosulae*, *Rhizoma Cimicifugae* and *Radix Bupleuri*.

3. Invigorate vital energy to strengthen the body; For common cold in debilitated patient, superficies-asthenia with profuse sweating, usually used to-

Commonly Used Drugs

gether with *Rhizoma Atractylodis Macrocephalae*.

4. Relieve skin infection and promote tissue regeneration: For unruptured abscess, unhealed carbuncle, skin erosion, unhealed wound, eruptive diseases and skin infection of *yin* type. Recently used for peptic ulcer and atrophic gastritis.

5. Promote diuresis and relieve edema: For edema of spleen-deficiency type. In addition, it can invigorate vital energy to promote the productionof body fluid and quench thirst and is indicated for diabetes; hemiplegia due to deficiency of vital energy and blood stasis. Also used for asthma and leukocytopenia.

Administration   Decoction: 9 – 15 g, up to 30 – 60 g.

Selected Recipes   For moisturizing skin:

Recipe 1: *Shengji huangqi wan*

Radix Astragali seu Hedysari	30 g
Herba Cistanchis	30 g
Radix Ginseng	30 g
Radix Ledebouriellae	30 g
Cortex Cinnamomi	30 g
Radix Platycodi	30 g
Rhizoma Achyranthis Bidentatae	30 g
Rhizoma Atractylodis Macrocephalae	30 g
Radix Paeoniae Alba	30 g
Poria	30 g
Radix Aconiti Praeparata	30 g

Grind the above drugs into fine powder and make it into honeyed pills. Each pill weighs about 1 g. Take 20 pills on an empty stomach each time.

Recipe 2: *Puji runfu fang*

Radix Astragali seu Hedysari	15 g
Radix Angelicae Sinensis	15 g
Radix Ledebouriellae	15 g
Lignum Santali Albi	15 g
Fructus Trichosanthis	15 g
Radix Angelicae Dahuricae	15 g
Radix Paeoniae Rubra	960 g

    Semen Armeniacae Amarum   960 g

Pound the drugs into pieces. Cook the dried drugs in a right amount of polished edible oil over a slow fire for 6 hours. Remove the dregs and cook the oil for another 6 hours. Store the filtered oil in a china pot for external use.

For pelade and grey hair:

Recipe: *Wantai baizhihuang gao*

Radix Astragali seu Hedysari	30 g
Radix Angelicae Sinensis	30 g
Radix Angelicae Pubescentis	30 g
Rhizoma Ligustici Chuanxiong	30 g
Radix Angelicae Dahuricae	30 g
Radix Paeoniae Alba	30 g
Radix Ledebouriellae	30 g
Flos Magnoliae	30 g
Bulbus Allii Macrostemi	15 g

Pound the drugs into pieces. Cook the dried drugs in a right amount of polished edible oil over a slow fire for 6 hours. Remove the dregs and cook the oil for another 6 hours. Store the filtered oil in a china pot for external use.

For pimples and freckles:

Recipe 1:

Radix Astragali seu Hedysari	75 g
Rhizoma Atractylodis Macrocephalae	75 g
Radix Cynanchi Atrati	75 g
Rhizoma Polygonati Odorati	45 g
Radix Phytolaccae	30 g
Radix Ledebouriellae	45 g
Rhizoma Ligustici Chuanxiong	45 g
Radix Angelicae Dahuricae	45 g
Herba Asari	45 g
Radix Aucklandiae	30 g
Semen Armeniacae Amarum	45 g
Rhizoma Typhonii	45 g

Grind the above drugs into fine powder except *Semen Armeniacae Amarum* which is ground into mash. Mix the powder and mash together and dry it in the sun. Apply a right amount of the mixture on the face at bedtime and wash it on the next morning.

Recipe 2:

Radix Astragali seu Hedysari	60 g
Rhizoma Atractylodis Macrocephalae	60 g
Radix Ampelopsis	60 g
Rhizoma Polygonati Odorati	60 g
Radix Trichosanthis	60 g
Radix Phytolaccae	60 g
Radix Ledebouriellae	60 g
Radix Angelicae Dahuricae	60 g
Herba Asari	60 g
Radix Aucklandiae	60 g
Rhizoma Typhonii	60 g
Rhizoma Ligustici Chuanxiong	60 g
Semen Armeniacae Amarum	60 g

Grind the above drugs into fine powder except *Semen Armeniacae Amarum* which is ground into mash. Mix the powder and mash together and dry it in the sun. Apply a right amount of the mixture on the face at bedtime and wash it on the next morning.

For leukodermia:

Recipe: Shishimilu baidianzidian fang

Frucus Xanthii	30 g
Radix Ledebouriellae	9 g
Radix Astragali seu Hedysari	90 g

Grind the above drugs into fine powder and make pills. Each pill weighs about 1 g. Take 3 pills before breakfast.

Caution   Contraindicated for cases with sthenic syndrome or syndrome of hyperactivity of *yang* and deficiency of *yin*.

Modern Research   30 g of *Radix Stephaniae Tetrandrae* and *Radix Astragali seu Hedysari* each, 15 g of prepared *Rhizoma Atractylodis Macrocephalae*, 6 g of *Radix Glycyrrhizae*, 9 g of *Rhizoma Zingiberis Recens*, 20 g of *Fructus Ziziphi Jujubae*, one dose daily. 12 cases with bromhidrosis were given the above treatment, all recovered completely.

Radix Angelicae Sinensis

Source Root of *Angelica sinensis* (Oliv.) Diels, family *Umbelliferae*.

Characteristics The axial root, conical, with several fibrous roots, 15 – 25 cm long, the root base 1.5 – 4.0 cm in diameter, brown in color. Cork longigudinally and transversely lenticellate; the root body longitudinally wrinkled; the root base rounded flat, with lanceolate stem leaf remnant lying flat at its top. Prepared by crosscutting, the section showing a broad cortex with brown spotted oil cavities and an even xylem, cambium ring appearing between them. Soft in texture, delicately fragrant in smell. Sweet and acrid in taste, warm in nature, and attributive to liver, heart and spleen meridians.

Indication 1. Enrich *blood*: For blood – deficiency syndrome, usually used together with *Radix Astragali seu Hedysari* (Decoction of of *Angelicae Sinensis* for Enriching Blood), or with *Radix Rehmanniae Praeparata* and *Radix Paeoniae Alba*.

2. Promote blood circulation, regulate menstruation and alleviate pain: For blood-deficiency, blood stasis or blood-dryness manifested by menoxenia, amenorrhea, menorrhagia; or marked by headache, chest pain, abdominal pain and rheumatism, usually used together with *Radix Salviae Miltiorrhizae*, *Olibanum*, and *Myrrha*; or manifested by the early stage of skin infection or unhealed skin lesions, urticaria, eczema, prurigo, leukoderma, apoplexy, prolapse of the rectum, bronchial asthma, arrhythmia, cor pulmonale, etc..

Moisturize dryness and loose bowel: For constipation attributive to dryness of the intestine and blood-deficiency.

Administration Decoction: 5 – 10 g.

Selected Recipes For moisturizing skin:

    Recipe: *Yangsheng jiu*

Radix Angelicae Sinensis	30 g
Arillus Longan	240 g
Fructus Lycii	120 g
Flos Chrysanthemi	30 g

Soak the above drugs in 4 liters of white spirit in a sealed jar for one month. Take right amount of spirit orally.

For shrunken skin:

Recipe: *Runzao yangrong tang*

Radix Angelicae Sinensis	6 g
Radix Rehmanniae	4 g
Radix Rehmanniae Praeparata	4 g
Radix Paeoniae Alba	4 g
Radix Gentianae Macrophyllae	4 g
Radix Scutellariae	4 g
Radix Ledebouriellae	3 g
Radix Glycyrrhizae	1 g

All the above drugs are to be decocted in water for oral administration.

For leukotrichia and odontoseisis:

Recipe 1: *Shengji danggui san*

Radix Angelicae Sinensis

crucian carp

Remove the internals of the crucian and fill it with powder of **Radix Angelicae Sinensis**. Heat the crucian until it has been carbonized. Brush teeth with the powder of the carbonized crucian and gargle the mouth as usual.

Recipe 2: *Jifeng danggui san*

Radix Angelicae Sinensis	30 g
Rhizoma Cyperi	36 g
Radix Rehmanniae	30 g
Radix Angelicae Dahuricae	30 g
edible salt	15 g
Fructus Gleditsiae	150 g
Radix Aconiti	60 g
Rhizoma Zingiberis Recens	150 g

Grind the above dried drugs into fine powder. Brush teeth with the powder of the carbonized crucian and gargle the mouth as usual.

Recipe 3: *Fushou danggui fang*

Radix Angelicae Sinensis	60 g
Rhizoma Ligustici Chuanxiong	60 g
Radix Rehmanniae Praeparata	60 g

Radix Paeoniae Alba	60 g
Rhizoma Cyperi	60 g
Fructus Lycii	60 g
Rhizoma Achyranthis Bidentatae	60 g
Herba Schizonepetae	60 g
edible salt	60 g

Grind the above dried drugs into fine powder. Brush teeth with the powder of the carbonized crucian and gargle the mouth as usual.

Recipe 4: *Wuxu guchi shenmiao san*

    Radix Angelicae Sinensis

    Radix Rehmanniae

    Flos Caryophylli

    edible salt

    Herba Ecliptae

    Herba Asari

    Gallae Turcicae

    Poria

Grind the above drugs into fine powder and take it as gargle and can be applied on grey hair.

For dandruff:

Recipe 1: *Mianyou mofeng gao*

Herba Ephedrae	6 g
Rhizoma Cimicifugae	6 g
Radix Ledebouriellae	6 g
Rhizoma seu Radix Notopterygii	3 g
Radix Angelicae Sinensis	3 g
Rhizoma Bletillae	3 g
Lignum Santali Albi	3 g

Decoct the drugs in polished oil over a slow fire. Then filter the dregs out. Add a right amount of vaseline in the oil and heat the oil until becomes some kind of ointment. Apply it on the scalp for one hour and clean the hair completely.

Recipe 2: *Fushou shensuo san*

    Radix Angelicae Sinensis

Commonly Used Drugs

    Radix Angelicae Dahuricae
    Semen Pharbitidis
    Fructus Chebulae
    Herba Schizonepetae
    Cacumen Biotae
    Radix Clematidis

Grind equal amount of the above drugs into fine powder. Apply it on the scalp and clean it up the next morning.

Caution   Contraindicated for cases with stagnation of dampness manifesting loose stools.

Modern Research   10 – 15 g of *Radix Angelicae Sinensis*, 15 – 20 g of *Radix Rehmanniae*, 10 – 12 g of *Rhizoma Ligustici Chuanxiong* and *Radix Paeoniae Rubra* each, 6 – 10 g of *Fructus Gardeniae* and *Flos Carthami* each, 3 g of *Resina Draconis*, 10 – 20 g of *Semen Dolichoris Albi* and *Bombyx Batryticatus* each, 10 g of *Rhizoma Typhonii* and *Radix Angelicae Dahuricae* each, 6 g of *deerhorn glue*, *Colla Corii Asini* and *Plastrum Testudinis*, decocted in water for oral administration, one dose daily. Decoct the dregs in 5000 ml of water until 3000 ml of decoction is obtained. Wash the affected area with the decoction for 30 minutes, then clean the skin with pure water, twice to three times daily. 33 cases with circumorbital birthmarks were given the above treatment, all improved, 21 cases got considerable curative effects.

    30 g of *Radix Angelicae Sinensis* and *Semen Coicis* each, 9 g of *Radix Paeoniae Rubra*, *Rhizoma Ligustici Chuanxiong*, *Rhizoma Ligustici Chuanxiong*, *Rhizoma Atractylodis Macrocephalae*, *Rhizoma Typhonii*, *Radix Angelicae Dahuricae*, *Radix Asparagi*, *Fructus Amomi* and *Radix Glycyrrhizae* each, 15 g of *Poria*, 12 g of *Rhizoma Polygonati Odorati*. *Radix Bupleuri* and *Rhizoma Cyperi* added for stagnation of liver-*qi*; *Semen Persicae*, *Flos Carthami* and *Herba Lycopi* added for *blood* stasis; *Cortex Moutan Radicis* and *Fructus Gardeniae* added for *blood*-heat; *Radix Codonopsis Pilosulae* and *Radix Astragali seu Hedysari* added for deficiency of *qi*; *Colla Corii Asini* and *Caulis Spatholobi* added for insufficiency of *blood*; *Rhizoma Atractylodis*, *Polyporus Umbellatus* and *Rhizoma Alismatis* added for stagnation of dampness; *Radix Aconiti Praeparata* and *Cortex Cinnamomi* added for *yang*-deficiency of kidney; *Radix Rehmanniae* and

Herba Dendrobii added for deficiency of kidney-*yin*, decocted in water for oral administration, one dose daily. Apply the decoction containing *Radix Ginseng*, *Radix Notoginseng*, *Flos Carthami* and *Radix Angelicae Sinensis* etc. on the affected part, twice to three times daily. 235 cases with moth-patches were given the above treatment. Among them 58 recovered completely, 69 improved considerably, 87 got some curative effect, 21 cases failed.

20 g of *Radix Angelicae Sinensis*, 10 g of *Rhizoma Ligustici Chuanxiong*, *Flos Carthami*, *Semen Persicae*, *Periostracum Cicadae*, *Radix Platycodi*, *Folium Eriobotryae*, *Fructus Tribuli* and *Rhizoma Cyperi* each, 15 g of *Radix Paeoniae Rubra*, 30 g of *Radix Rehmanniae*, 5 g of *Radix Glycyrrhizae*, decocted in water for oral administration, one dose daily. 10 cases with moth-patches were given the above treatment. Among them, 8 recovered completely, one improved, one failed. The course of disease ranging from one month to one year and a half.

Semen Coicis

Source The dried mature seed of *Coix lacryma-jobi* L. var. ma-yuen (Roman.) Stapf, family *Gramineae*.

Characteristics Seed spheroidal or semi-spherical, obtuse-round at one end and somewhat flat at the other, 0.5 – 0.7 cm in length. Surface smooth, milky white in color, occasionally remained with brownish testa. A deeply and widely grooved, concavely basilar and spotted hilum appearing at the flat end. Hard in texture. Fracture section appearing white and farinaceous. Sweet and bland in taste, slightly cold in nature, and attributive to spleen, stomach, lung and large intestine meridians.

Indication 1. Promote diuresis and invigorate the spleen: For spleen-deficiency syndrome with accumulation of dampness manifested by edema, beriberi, or diarrhea; for stranguria of dampness-heat type and of stone origin; for dampness febrile disease manifested by fever, bodily heaviness, oppressive sensation over the chest and epigastrium, anorexia, and smooth or greasy tongue coating.

2. Relieve dampness obstruction and relax the muscles: For arthralgia of

Commonly Used Drugs

wind-dampness type and muscular rigidity.

3. Clear away heat to drain the pus: For lung abscess, usually used together with *Rhizoma Phragmitis*, *Semen Benincasae* and *Semen Persicae*; for appendicitis, usually used together with *Herba Patriniae*, *Semen Persicae* and *Cortex Mori Radicis*.

Administration Decoction: 10 – 30 g.

Selected Recipes For flat wart:

  Recipe:

Semen Gingko	8 – 12
Semen Coicis	60 g

Decoct the drugs in a right amount of water until it is done. Add a right amount of white sugar and mix it well. Take the mixture orally.

For flat wart, acne, and freckles:

  Recipe:

Semen Coicis	30 g
Bulbus Lillii	6 g

Decoct the drugs in a right amount of water until it is done. Add a right amount of white sugar and mix it well. Take the mixture on an empty stomach, once in the morning and once in the evening.

Caution Contraindicated for pregnant women.

Modern Research 60 g of *Semen Coicis* and a right amount of rice done as gruel, take it once daily. 23 cases of flat wart were given the above treatment. Among them, 11 fully recovered, 6 improved, 6 failed. The cource of treatment ranges from 7 to 16 days. 60 g of *Semen Coicis*, 8 g of *Herba Ephedrae* and *Radix Glycyrrhizae* each, 10 g of *Semen Armeniacae Amarum*. *Radix Astragali seu Hedysari* added for *qi*-deficiency; *Radix Angelicae Sinensis* added for *blood*-deficiency; *Rhizoma Atractylodis Macrocephalae* and *Pericarpium Citri Reticulatae* added for deficiency of spleen; *Bombyx Batryticatus* added for hard surface of the wart, decocted in water for oral administration, one dose daily. 20 cases of flat wart were given the above treatment. All recovered after the treatment.

  Recipe: *Chuyou tang*

Semen Coicis	30 g
Folium Isatidis	30 g

Radix Isatidis	30 g
Concha Ostreae	30 g
Herba Patriniae	15 g
Spica Prunellae	15 g
Radix Paeoniae Rubra	10 g

All the above drugs are to be decocted in water for oral administration. Decoct the dregs and wash the affected part with the filtered decoction. One course of treatment consists of 7 days. 50 cases of flat wart were given the above treatment. Among them, 35 recovered completely, 12 improved considerably, 3 failed after 5 courses of treatment.

50 g of *Semen Coicis* and *Gypsum Fibrosum* each, 15 g of *Herba Ephedrae*, *Semen Armeniacae Amarum* and *Radix Ledebouriellae* each, 10 g of *Radix Glycyrrhizae*, 20 g of *Rhizoma Ligustici Chuanxiong*, *Radix Rehmanniae* and *Radix Paeoniae Rubra* each, one dose once other day. 300 cases with acne were given the above treatment. All recovered after 3 – 12 months of treatment. The course of treatment averages 6 months.

Cortex Lycii Radicis

Source   The root cortex of *Lycium chinensis* Mill. and *L. barbarum* L., family *Solanaceae*.

Characteristics   The root cortex quilled or groove – shaped, unequal in length, 0.5 – 1.5 cm broad, 0.1 – 0.3 cm thick; epidermis grey-yellow, easily exfoliating; endodermis yellow-white to grey-white, with fine longitudinal striae. Light in weight and fragile. Section unsmooth, yellow at the surface and white inside. Bitter and bland in taste, cold in nature, and attributive to lung and kidney meridians.

Indication   1. Lower asthenic fever: For fever due to *yin*-deficiency and the late stage of febrile disease with *yin*-consumption, manifested by fever high at night and subsided in the morning, hectic fever, night sweat, red and dry tongue without fur, etc., and for infantile malnutrition with fever, usually used together with *Rhizoma Anemarrhenae*, *Carapax Trionycis*, etc..

Commonly Used Drugs

2. Clear away heat and cool the *blood*: For hematemesis, epistaxis, hemoptysis and hematuria due to blood-heat.

3. Clear away lung-heat: For cough and dyspnea due to lung-heat, usually used together with *Cortex Mori Radicis*, *Radix Glycyrrhizae*, *Fructus Oryzae Sativae* (Powder for Expelling Lung-Heat).

4. Lower blood pressure: For hypertension. In addition, also for tuberculosis lymphadenitis, urticaria, allergic purpura, drug rash, allergy to insect bite, etc..

Administration Decoction: 6–12 g.

Selected Recipes For darkening grey hair and improving complexion:

Recipe 1:

Cortex Lycii Radicis	4,800 g
Radix Rehmanniae	1,200 g

Grind the above drugs into fine powder. Take 30 g orally each time.

Recipe 2:

Cortex Lycii Radicis	480 g
Radix Rehmanniae	480 g
Fructus Rubi	480 g

Grind the above drugs into fine powder. Make it into honeyed pills. Each weighs about 1 g. Take 40 pills on an empty stomach.

Recipe 3:

Cortex Lycii Radicis	150 g
Radix Rehmanniae	150 g
Rhizoma Achyranthis Bidentatae	90 g
Fructus Rubi	90 g
Radix Astragali seu Hedysari	90 g
Fructus Schisandrae	90 g
Semen Persicae	120 g
Semen Cuscutae	120 g
Fructus Tribuli	120 g

Grind the above drugs into fine powder. Make it into honeyed pills. Each weighs about 1 g. Take 40 pills with warm gruel on an empty stomach.

Recipe 4:

Cortex Lycii Radicis	300 g

Radix Rehmanniae Praeparata	300 g
Fructus Chebulae	60 g
Radix Angelicae Dahuricae	60 g
Cortex Cinnamomi	60 g
Semen Armeniacae Amarum	60 g
Pericarpium Zanthoxyli	60 g
Flos Inulae	30 g

Grind the above drugs into fine powder. Make it into honeyed pills. Each weighs about 1 g. Take 50 pills with warm millet on an empty stomach.

For odontolithiasis:

Recipe: *Digupi san*

Cortex Lycii Radicis	30 g
Semen Pruni	30 g
Radix Rehmanniae	30 g
Semen Armeniacae Amarum	30 g
Rhizoma Cimicifugae	45 g
Rhizoma Ligustici	15 g
Nidus Vespae	15 g

Grind the above drugs into fine powder. Take 3 g of such powder as gargle.

For halitosis:

Recipe:

Cortex Lycii Radicis
Cortex Mori Radicis
Radix Astragali seu Hedysari
Fructus Gardeniae
Fructus Aristolochiae
Radix Glycyrrhizae

All the above drugs decocted in water. One half of the warm decoction taken as gargle, another half for drinking.

For decayed teeth, odontoseisis and gingivitis:

Recipe: *Yuchi san*

Cortex Lycii Radicis
Radix Angelicae Dahuricae

Rhizoma Cimicifugae
Radix Ledebouriellae
Herba Asari
Rhizoma Ligustici Chuanxiong
Flos Sophorae
Radix Angelicae Sinensis
Rhizoma Ligustici
Radix Glycyrrhizae

Grind equal amount of the above drugs into fine powder. Brush the teeth with the powder. Decoct 6 g of the powder. Take the filtered decoction as gargle.

For bromidrosis:

Recipe:

Cortex Lycii Radicis	15 g
Cortex Mori Radicis	15 g
Radix Phytolaccae	30 g
Fructus Piperis Nigri	30 g
Talci	30 g

Grind the above drugs into fine powder. Mix it with white spirit and apply it on the affected part.

Caution Contraindicated for cases with syndrome of deficiency of stomach-*yang*.

Modern Research

Recipe:

Cortex Lycii Radicis
Cortex Dictamni Radicis
Cortex Moutan Radicis
Radix Rehmanniae
Radix Paeoniae Rubra
Radix Angelicae Sinensis
Rhizoma Ligustici Chuanxiong
Rhizoma Achyranthis Bidentatae

Cortex Phellodendri, **Rhizoma Atractylodis** and **Semen Coicis** added for dampness stagnation; **Radix Ledebouriellae** and **Periostracum Cicadae**

added for wind-evil. Decocted in water for oral administration. The treatment begins 12 to 15 days after menstruation, one dose daily, one course consisting of 6 to 9 days. Three courses recommended. 88 cases with female acne were given the above treatment, 61 improves considerably, 24 received some curative effects, 3 failed.

Radix Rehmanniae

Source Root of *Rehmannia glutinosa* Libosch., family *Scrophulariaceae*.

Characteristics The root appearing as irregular masses or flat-twisted strips, unequal in size; surface grey-black, wrinkled and striated. Section appearing black, lustrous, even and without striae. Heavy in weight and soft in texture. Sweet in taste, cold in nature, and attributive to heart, liver and kidney meridians.

Indication Clear away heat and cool the *blood*, nourish *yin* to promote the productionof bodyly fluid: For (1) seasonal febrile diseases involving yingfen and xuefen, manifested by fever and irritability; (2) blood-heat syndrome manifested by hematemesis, epistaxis, hemoptysis, eruptions, hematuria, hemafecia, metrorrhagia, etc.; (3) febrile diseases with consumption of bodyly fluid manifested by fever, thirst and constipation; (4) syndrome of *yin*-deficiency and fire-hyperactivity with hectic fever; (5) lung-dryness syndrome with cough or epistaxis; (6) sthenic or asthenic heat-syndrome with sorethroat; (7) diabetes.

Administration Decoction: 9 – 30 g.

Selected Recipes See those in *Radix Rehmanniae Praeparata*.

Modern Research See those in *Radix Rehmanniae Praeparata*.

Radix Rehmanniae Praeparata

Source Root of *Rehmannia glutinosa* Libosch., family *Scrophulariaceae*. Prepared by steaming it with wine and drying repeatedly.

Characteristics Root irregular masses, vaying in size, dark and lustrous. Soft and sticky in texture. Sweet and slightly bitter in taste, slightly warm in nature, and attributive to heart, liver and kidney meridians.

Indication 1. Produce essence and enrich blood: For insufficiency of essence and blood manifested by sallow complexion, fatigue, dizziness, palpitation, menoxenia and metrorrhagia.

2. Nourish *yin* and moisturize dyness: For deficiency of liver-*yin* and kidney-*yin* manifested by hectic fever, night sweat, emission and diabetes, usually used together with **Fructus Corni** and **Rhizoma Dioscoreae**; also used for prurigo due to dryness of *blood*, muscular spasm due to *blood*-deficiency or *yin*-deficiency, and constipation due to insufficiency of bodily fluid and *blood*.

3. Invigorate the liver and kidney: For backache with knee aching due to deficiency of liver and kidney, such as chronic lumbar strain, hyperplasia of lumbar vertebra, etc.; for endemic osteoarthritis deformans, usually used together with **Herba Cistanchis**; also for dyspnea and chronic cough of kidney-deficiency type. Recently used singly for hypertensionand hypercholesterinemia.

Administration Decoction: 10 – 30 g

Selected Recipes For darkening grey hair and moisturizing skin:

  Recipe 1:

Radix Rehmanniae Praeparata	150 g
Rhizoma Achyranthis Bidentatae	120 g
Semen Armeniacae Amarum	60 g
Semen Cuscutae	90 g

Grind the above drugs into fine powder and make it into honeyed pills. Each weighs about 1 g. Take 30 pills at bedtime.

  Recipe 2: *Shengji xiaodihuang jian*

Radix Rehmanniae	4800 g
deerhorn glue	480 g
Fructus Perillae	600 g
Rhizoma Zingiberis Recens	150 g
Mel	2 liters
white spirit	4 liters

Grind **Radix Rehmanniae**, **Rhizoma Zingiberis Recens** and **Fructus Perillae** to get juice. Decoct the glue and honey in the juice and white spirits until deerhorn glue is dissolved. Store the decoction in a sealed chinese jar. Take one spoon each time.

Recipe 3: *Er huang wan*

Radix Rehmanniae	30 g
Radix Rehmanniae Praeparata	30 g
Radix Asparagi	30 g
Radix Ophiopogonis	30 g
Radix Ginseng	30 g

Grind the above drugs into fine powder and make it into honeyed pills. Each weighs about 1 g. Take 30 pills with warm millet wine on an empty stomach.

Recipe 4: *Qiongyu gao*

Radix Rehmanniae	8000 g
Radix Ginseng	150 g
Poria	1600 g
Mel	4800 g

Grind *Radix Rehmanniae* to get juice. Decoct other drugs in the juice over a slow fire for 10 hours. Take one spoon each time.

For invigorating kidney to improve complexion:

Recipe 1: *Zengyi bawei wan*

Radix Rehmanniae Praeparata	120 g
Cornu Cervi Pantotrichi	120 g
Fructus Schisandrae	120 g
Rhizoma Dioscoreae	60 g
Fructus Corni	60 g
Radix Aconiti Praeparata	60 g
Rhizoma Achyranthis Bidentatae	60 g
Poria	45 g
Cortex Moutan Radicis	45 g
Rhizoma Alismatis	45 g

Grind the above drugs along with 150 g of deehorn glue into fine powder and make it into honeyed pills. Each weighs about 1 g. Take 30 pills with millet on an empty stomach.

Recipe 2:

Radix Rehmanniae	a right amount
Mel	a right amount

Grind *Radix Rehmanniae* to get juice. Decoct honey in the juice until the decoction become extracted. Make the extract into pills. Each weighs about 1 g. Take 30 pills each time.

For calvities and sallow complexion:

Recipe:

Radix Rehmanniae Praeparata	30 g
Radix Angelicae Sinensis	30 g
Cornu Cervi Pantotrichi	60 g

Grind the above drugs into fine powder and make it into honeyed pills. Each weighs about 1 g. Take 50 pills with rice gruel.

For darkening grey hair:

Recipe 1:

Radix Rehmanniae	2.5 kg
Cortex Acanthopanacis Radicis	150 g
Rhizoma Achyranthis Bidentatae	150 g

Soak *Radix Rehmanniae* in white spirits for 48 hours. Grind the above drugs into fine powder and take 6 g with warm millet on an empty stomach.

Recipe 2:

Radix Rehmanniae	1 kg
Radix Rubiae	0.5 kg

Grind *Radix Rehmanniae* to get juice. Decoct *Radix Rubiae* in 2.5 liters of water over a slow fire for 5 minutes. Then extract *Radix Rubiae* to get juice. Mix the juice of the two drugs and heat them over a slow fire until extract is got. Take one spoon on an empty stomach.

Recipe 3:

Succus Rehmanniae	one liter
Succus Zingiberis Recens	500 ml
Fructus Piperis Nigri	30 g
Radix Rehmanniae Praeparata	30 g
Flos Inulae	30 g
Fructus Mori	30 g

Decoct the juice until it is done. Grind the other drugs into fine powder and make it into honeyed pills with the juice. Each weighs about 6 g. Take one pill in the mouth and swallow the dissolved.

Recipe 4:

Radix Rehmanniae	480 g
Fructus Rubi	480 g
Cortex Lycii Radicis	480 g

Grind the above drugs into fine powder and make it into honeyed pills. Each weighs about 1 g. Take 40 pills with warm millet wine on an empty stomach.

For odontoseisis:

Recipe 1:

Radix Rehmanniae	2 kg
Rhizoma Dioscoreae	120 g
Radix Ginseng	120 g
Cortex Lycii Radicis	90 g
Poria	120 g

Grind *Radix Rehmanniae* to get juice. Grind the other drugs into fine powder and decoct it in 10 liters of white spirits until 3 liters remained. Remove the dregs and add the juice of *Radix Rehmanniae* and 0.5 kg of honey. Decoct the mixture until it becomes some kind of extract. Make pills with it, each weighs about 1 g. Take 20 pills each time, three times daily.

Recipe 2:

Radix Rehmanniae	60 g
Fructus Tribuli	60 g
Rhizoma Cyperi	120 g
Gallae Turcicae	30 g
Fructus Psoraleae	60 g
edible salt	30 g

Grind the above drugs into fine powder. Brush teeth with the powder. Take 10 g additionally prior to breakfast.

For gingivitis:

Recipe:

Radix Rehmanniae	0.5 kg

Commonly Used Drugs

Moschus	0.3 g
edible salt	50 g

Grind the above drugs into fine powder and apply it on the affected part.

For odontoseisis and grey hair:

Recipe: *Yi ya san*

Radix Rehmanniae Praeparata	60 g
Cortex Lycii Radicis	60 g
Rhizoma Ligustici Chuanxiong	60 g
edible salt	60 g
Rhizoma Cyperi	60 g
Fructus Psoraleae	60 g
Herba Asari	8 g
Radix Ledebouriellae	8 g
Fructus Tribuli	15 g
Cortex Acanthopanacis Radicis	15 g
Gypsum Fibrosum	15 g
Pericarpium Zanthoxyli	6 g
Fructus Gleditsiae	

powder and brush teeth with it. In addition, take 6 g orally once daily.

For herpes facialis:

Recipe:

Radix Rehmanniae	1.2 kg
Cortex Lycii Radicis	4.8 kg

Grind the above drugs into fine powder and take 10 g on an empty stomach.

For acne rosacea:

Recipe: *Jingui gouxuan fang*

Radix Rehmanniae

Flos Chrysanthemi

Rhizoma Ligustici Chuanxiong

Radix Angelicae Sinensis

Pericarpium Citri Reticulatae

Flos Carthami

Radix Scutellariae

Faeces Trogopterori

Decoct the first seven drugs until they are done. Add the powder of *Faeces Trogopterori* in the filtered decoction and take one dose daily.

Modern Research 180 g of *Radix Rehmanniae*, 150 g of *Radix Rehmanniae Praeparata*, *Fructus Ligustri Lucidi* and *Radix Angelicae Sinensis* each, 225 g of *Cacumen Biotae*, 7.5 of *Rhizoma seu Radix Notopterygii*. Grind the above drugs into fine powder. Take 6 - 9 g with warm water each time, three times daily. Also can be made into capsules. Soak 9 g of *Cacumen Biotae* in 700 ml of 75% alcohol in a sealed bottle for 7 - 10 days. Apply a right amount of the filtered tincture on the affected part to and fro for 10 minutes, three times daily. The above treatment were given to 86 cases with alopecia areata. Among them, 62 recovered completely, 18 improved, 6 failed. 16 cases revealed recurrence at follow-ups.

12 g of *Radix Rehmanniae*, *Radix Rehmanniae*, *Radix Polygoni Multiflori Praeparata* and *Fructus Tribuli* each, decocted in water for oral administration, one dose daily. One course of treatment consists of two months. 30 g of *Fructus Psoraleae* and 1 g of sulfur and oxybenzoic acid is soaked in 100 ml of 75% alcohol for 3 to 7 days. The tincture is applied on the thin skin of the affected part. 30 g of *Fructus Psoraleae*, 10 g of sulfur and 6 g of oxybenzoic acid is soaked in 100 ml of 95% alcohol for 3 to 7 days. The tincture is applied on the thick skin of the affected part. Rub the skin until it is congested. Sun bathing is applied 10 to 30 minutes. The above treatment was given to 50 cases of leukodermia. Of them, 15 fully recovered, 26 improved, 9 failed.

Herba Asari

Source Herb of *Asarum heterotropoides* Fr. Schmidt var. *mandshuricum* (Maxim.) Kitag. and *A. sieboldii* Miq., family *Aristolochiaceae*.

Characteristics Herb. Rhizome slender, nodose, with many slender fibrous roots at the nodes. Basal leaves with long petiole, blades cordate. With pungent and fragrant odor. Acrid in taste, warm in nature, and attributive to lung and kidney meridians.

Indication 1. Induce sweating to expel cold and exogenous evils from the body surface, expel wind and relieve pain: For common cold of wind-cold type with severe headache and general aching, especially for the case with *yang*-deficiency, recurrent headache, headache of wind-cold type, toothache, arthralgia of wind-cold-dampness type.

2. Warm the lung to promote expectoration: For cough and dyspnea with thin sputum attributive to lung-cold.

3. Wake up from unconsciousness: For sudden syncope, use powder for nasal insufflation to induce sneezing.

Administration Decoction: 1 – 3 g.

Selected Recipes For odontoseisis:

Recipe: *Jingyue xuanfeng laoya san*

Herba Asari	21 g
Radix Angelicae Sinensis	30 g
Rhizoma Ligustici Chuanxiong	30 g
edible salt	21 g

Grind the above drugs into fine powder. Brush teeth with the powder. Take 6 g orally in the capsule, once daily.

For dim complexion:

Recipe 1:

Herba Asari	3 g
Rhizoma Polygonati Odorati	3 g
Radix Astragali seu Hedysari	3 g
Rhizoma Typhonii	3 g
Rhizoma Dioscoreae	3 g
Flos Magnoliae	3 g
Rhizoma Ligustici Chuanxiong	3 g
Radix Angelicae Dahuricae	3 g
Fructus Trichosanthis	6 g
Cortex Magnoliae	6 g

Decoct the above drugs in a right amount of water. Wash face with the decoction. Clean it half one hour later.

Recipe 2:

Os Sepiella seu Sepiae	60 g
Herba Asari	60 g

Fructus Trichosanthis	60 g
Rhizoma Zingiberis	60 g
Pericarpium Zanthoxyli	60 g

Soak the drugs in white spirits for 3 days. Decoct the drugs and tincture until alcohol is volatilized. Wash face with the warm decoction. Clean it half one hour later.

For calvities:

Recipe: *Waitai shengfa gao*

Herba Asari	40 g
Radix Ledebouriellae	40 g
Radix Dipsaci	40 g
Rhizoma Ligustici Chuanxiong	40 g
Fructus Gleditsiae	40 g
Cacumen Biotae	40 g
Flos Magnoliae	40 g
Ramulus Loranthis	75 g
Herba Lycopi	80 g
Fructus Viticis	120 g
Succus Mori Radicis	one liter
Bulbus Allii Macrostemi	120 g
Folium Bambusae	90 g
Folium Pini	90 g
Radix Angelicae Dahuricae	180 g

Soak the above drugs in a right amount of white spirits for 12 hours. Filter the tincture and apply it on the affected part, twice to three times daily.

For grey hair and odontoseisis:

Recipe: *Caya san*

Herba Asari
Rhizoma Ligustici Chuanxiong
Semen Nelumbinis
Rhizoma Cyperi
Radix Rehmanniae
Radix Angelicae Sinensis

Heat the drugs until they are carbonized. Grind them into fine powder.

Commonly Used Drugs

Brush teeth with the powder and take 6 g orally, once daily.

For foul breath:

Recipe 1:

    Herba Asari

    Fructus Amomi Rotundus

Hold the drugs in mouth.

Recipe 2: *Shengji xixin san*

Herba Asari	1 g
Rhizoma Acori Calami	2 g
Rhizoma Zingiberis	15 g
Fructus Ziziphi Jujubae	15 g
Ligni Aquilariae	0.5 g

Grind the above drugs into fine powder. Hold 3 g of the powder in mouth in order to increase salivation. Swallow the saliva.

For odontoseisis and pararhisoclasia.

Recipe: *Shenghui xixin san*

Herba Asari	60 g
Rhizoma Cimicifugae	60 g
Cortex Lycii Radicis	60 g
Herba Artemisiae Annuae	60 g
Rhizoma Achyranthis Bidentatae	90 g
Radix Rehmanniae	150 g

Grind the carbonized drugs into fine powder. Apply it on the affected part at bedtime, gargle mouth in the next morning.

Recipe: *Jufang xixin san*

Herba Asari	30 g
Herba Schizonepetae	30 g
Pericarpium Zanthoxyli	15 g
Fructus Carpesii Abrotanoidis	15 g
Fructus Gleditsiae	15 g
Fructus Piperis Longi	15 g
Fructus Amomi	15 g
Radix Angelicae Dahuricae	60 g
Radix Aconiti	60 g

Grind the above drugs into fine powder. Brush teeth with the powder. Swallowing prohibited. Gargle mouth with clean water after the treatment.

For dental plaques:

Recipe: Shengji xixin san

Herba Asari	1 g
Rhizoma Cimicifugae	1 g
Rhizoma Ligustici	1 g
Rhizoma Ligustici Chuanxiong	1 g
Radix Ledebouriellae	1 g
Radix Glycyrrhizae	1 g
Gypsum Lamelliforme	15 g

Grind the above drugs into fine powder. Apply the powder on the teeth at bedtime and clean the mouth the next morning.

Fructus Lycii

Source Fruit of *Lycium barbarum* L., family *Solanaceae*.

Characteristics Fruit nearly cambiform, 6 – 18 mm long. Carpodermis red, wrinkled, soft, smooth and sticky, containing many flat reniform seeds. Sweet in taste, mild in nature, and attributive to liver and kidney meridians.

Indication Nourish *yin*, enrich *blood*, benefit essence and improve visual acuity: For deficiency of liver-*yin* and kidney-*yin* and insufficiency of essence and blood manifested by dizziness, blurring of vision, hypopsia, tinnitus, emission and soreness of the loin and extremities; also for diabetes.

Administration Decoction: 6 – 15 g.

Selected Recipes For invigorating primordial vital energy, moisturizing skin and improving complexion:

Recipe: Shengji gouqi wan

Fructus Lycii	300 g
Flos Chrysanthemi	120 g
Cortex Cinnamomi	45 g
Poria	30 g
Radix Rehmanniae Praeparata	30 g

Commonly Used Drugs

  Succus Menthae   20 ml

Grind the first four drugs into fine powder and make it into honeyed pills with the juice of peppermint. Each weighs about 1 g. Take 20 pills with millet wine on an empty stomach.

  Recipe: *Shengji gouqi jian*

Succus Lycii	3 liters
Succus Rehmanniae	3 liters
Succus Ophiopogonis	250 ml
Semen Armeniacae Amarum	150 g
Radix Ginseng	90 g
Poria	90 g

Grind *Radix Ginseng* and *Poria* into fine powder. Grind *Semen Armeniacae Amarum* into mash. Decoct the first four ingredients over slow fire until thin gruel is got. Add the powder of *Radix Ginseng* and *Poria* in the gruel and continue cooking until the gruel is extracted enough. Take half one spoon of the extract with millet wine each time, twice daily.

  For darkening grey hair:

  Recipe: *Dixian wan*

Fructus Lycii	60 g
Massa Fermentata Medicinalis	60 g
Flos Chrysanthemi	60 g
Radix Rehmanniae Praeparata	60 g
Cortex Cinnamomi	60 g
Herba Cistanchis	45 g

Grind the above drugs into fine powder and make it into honeyed pills. Each weighs about 1 g. Take 30 pills with millet wine on an empty stomach.

  For moisturizing skin and longevity:

  Recipe: *Shengji gouqizi wan*

Fructus Lycii	30 g
Fructus Rubi	30 g
Semen Plantaginis	30 g
Radix Rehmanniae	30 g
Cortex Lycii Radicis	30 g
Radix Dipsaci	30 g

Radix Polygoni Multiflori	30 g
Radix Morindae Officinalis	30 g
Flos Chrysanthemi	30 g
Rhizoma Atractylodis Macrocephalae	30 g
Rhizoma Acori Calami	30 g
Radix Polygalae	30 g
Herba Asari	30 g
Rhizoma Achyranthis Bidentatae	30 g
Semen Cuscutae	30 g

Grind the above drugs into fine powder and make it into honeyed pills. Each weighs about 1 g. Take 15 to 20 pills on an empty stomach.

For facial vesicles:

Recipe: *Shenghui gouqizi san*

Fructus Lycii	30 g
Poria	30 g
Semen Armeniacae Amarum	30 g
Radix Ledebouriellae	30 g
Herba Asari	30 g
Radix Angelicae Dahuricae	30 g

Grind the above drugs into fine powder and decoct it in a right amount of water for a while. Wash the face with the decoction. Clean it one hour later.

Caution Contraindicated for cases with sthenic heat evil and dampness stagnation in the spleen meridian manifesting diarrhea.

Semen Persicae

Source The seed of *Prunus persica* (L.) Batsch and *P. davidiana* Franch., family *Rosaceae*.

Characteristics Seed flat-ovate or nearly elliptical, 1.2 – 2.0 cm long; apex acute, base obliquely round, perine thin. Spermoderm yellow-brown, with a round chalaza at the base, and a linear hilum at the top, numerous vascular bundles running longitudinally from the chalaza, and slightly branching reticularly. Bitter and sweet in taste, mild in nature, and attributive to lung, liver and large intestine meridians.

Indication 1. Promote blood circulation, remove blood stasis and relieve carbuncle: For blood-stasis syndrome with amenorrhea, dysmenorrhea and abdominal mass. Recently, used for hysteromyoma, used together with *Ramulus Cinnamomi*, *Poria*, *Cortex Mori Radicis*, *Radix Paeoniae Rubra* (Bolus of *Ramulus Cinnamomi* and *Poria*). Also for traumata, especially the injury of the chest, abdomen and spine; for acute appendicitis, used together with *Radix et Rhizoma Rhei*, *Cortex Mori Radicis*, etc.; for pulmonay abscess, used together with *Rhizoma Phragmitis*, *Semen Coicis*, etc.. Recently, injections are used for central retinitis, pigmentary degerneration of retina, postocular optic neuritis, optic atrophy, etc..

2. Relieve cough and asthma.

3. Promote blood circulation and moisturize dryness: For blood-stasis and *blood* dryness with pruitic eruptions.

Moisturize the intestine and relax the bowels: For constipation due to dryness of the intestine.

Administration Decoction: 6 – 12 g (crushed before decocting). The spermoderm should be retained for when being used for asthma.

Selected Recipes For smoothing facial skin:

Recipe: *Shenghui fang*

Semen Persicae	300 g
Fructus Viticis	300 g
Rhizoma Atractylodis Macrocephalae	180 g
Radix Trichosanthis	210 g
Fructus Piperis Longi	360 g

Grind the above drugs into fine powder or mash. Decoct it in a right amount of water for a while. Wash the face with the decoction.

For smoothing skin of the hand:

Recipe: *Qianjin yi fang*

Semen Persicae	60 g
Semen Armeniacae Amarum	60 g
Semen Citri Reticulatae	20 g
Semen Phaseoli	10 g
Flos Magnoliae	30 g

Rhizoma Ligustici Chuanxiong	30 g
Radix Angelicae Sinensis	30 g
Fructus Ziziphi Jujubae	20
beef brain	60 g
mutton brain	60 g
dog brain	60 g

Soak the ingredients in 7 liters of white spirits for one day. Decoct the mixture over a slow fire for one hour. Filter out the dregs and continue cooking the decoction until it is extracted enough. Clean up the hands with pure water. Then apply the extract on the hands. Keep away from fire.

For leukoderma:

Recipe: *Shenghui fang*

Semen Persicae	150 g
Semen Sesami	400 g
Radix Rehmanniae	150 g

Grind the above drugs into fine powder and take 9 g each time, twice daily.

Modern Research 6 g of *Semen Persicae* and *Semen Armeniacae Amarum* each, 3 g of *Semen Chaulmoograe*, 10 g of *Semen Cannabis*, 3 g of *Hydrargyrum*. Grind the first four drugs into mash and mix it with mercury thoroughly. Wrapped with a piece of gauze. Rub the affected part with the medicated gauze for 3 to 5 minutes, three times daily. Store the gauze in a sealed container. The medicated gauze can be used for 10 days. One course of treatment consists of one month. 50 cases with acne rosacea were given the above treatment. Among them, 35 recovered completely, 9 got considerable curative effect, 5 improved in some degree, one failed. Oral administration prohibited. Prohibited for pregnant women.

Caution Contraindicated for pregnant women.

Part Three
Commonly Used Prescriptions

Anti-inflammatory and Analgesic Bolus
(Pian Zi Huang)

Ingredients

Not yet published. 0.3 g each piece, or slice, 0.6 g each packet.

Administration and Dosage

To be taken orally, children: 1 – 8 years, 0.15 – 0.3 g; over 8 years and adults, 0.6 g each time. Twice or three times a day. External Use, for original appearance of black or white vesiculae of innominate inflammatory swelling, mix one or two slices of *Pian Zi Huang* with cold boiled water or vinegar and apply it to the affected area; in case of ulceration, apply it to the perripheral area several times a day to keep local dampness.

Efficacy

Clearing away heat and toxic materials, relieving swelling and pain.

Indications

Acute or chronic hepatitis, tympanitis, gum abscess, oral ulcer, bee sting, snakebite, nail-like boil and innominate inflammatory swelling.

Anti-inflammatory Pill
(Liu Ying Wan)

Ingredients

Margarita
Calculus Bovis
Venenum Bufonis
Pills, 100 pills per bottle.

Efficacy

Clearing away heat and toxic material, subduing swelling and pain.

Indications

Tonsillitis, furuncle, sore, diseases of throat, the bite of insects, etc..

Administration and Dosage

To be taken orally with boiled water. Adults: 10 pills each time; children: 5 pills each time; infants: 2 pills each time, 3 times a day.

For external use, disintegrate some pills in just a little cold boiled water or vinegar and then apply it to the affected part of skin.

Cautions

Never to be administered to pregnant women.

Acanthopanax Infusion
(Wujiashen Chongji)

Ingredients

Radix Acanthopanacis Senticosi

Process

Make medicinal cubes (infusion), 25 g each cube.

Actions

Strengthening the body resistance and restoring normal functions of the body to consolidate the constitution, relieving mental stress and promoting intelligence.

Indications

Insomnia, excessive dreadming, fatigue and weakness, poor appetite and others caused by neurosis and other diseases. It has certain effects in relieving angina pectoris of coronary heart disease. It is also used for the treatment of leukopenia.

Direction

To be taken orally after being infused in boiling water, one cube eahc time, twice daily.

Banlong Pill
(Ban Long Wan)

Ingredients

Colla Cornu Cervi	10 g
Poria	10 g
Semen Biotae	10 g
Semen Cuscutae	10 g
Fructus Psoraleae	10 g
Pulvis Cornu Cervi	20 g
Radix Rehmanniae Praeparata	20 g

Efficacy

Nourishing and invigorating the kidney-essence, preserving sperm and tranquilizing; mainly for cases of nocturnal emission, impotence or premature ejaculation accompanied with lumbago, tinnitus, nocturia, dizziness, fatigue, pale complexion, pale tongue with white fur, sunken and small, weak pulse, which are attributive to the impairment of kidney-essence and weakness of kidney qi.

Indications

1. Applicable to cases of prolonged metrorrhagia or leucorrhagia, accompanied with dizziness, lumbago, weakness of the knee joints, spiritlessness, pale tongue with whitish fur, feeble pulse, which are attributive to insufficiency of essential substance and blood and weakness of kidney qi.

2. For cases with spontaneous flow of thin breast milk after delivery, shortness of breath, fatigue, lumbago, dimmish complexion, pale tongue with whitish fur, sunken and feeble pulse, which are attributive to insufficiency of kidney-essence and deficiency of kidney qi.

3. Also applicable to cases of hypothyroidism, neurasthenia, Addison's disease, dysfunctional uterine bleeding, hysteromyoma and endometritis, which are attributive to insufficiency of essential substance and blood, and deficiency of kid-

ney qi.

Interpretation

Colla Cornu Cervi not only invigorates essential substance and blood but also warms and strengthens kidney yang, and serves as the principal drug of the prescription. Radix Rehmanniae Praeparata and Semen Cuscutae can benefit yin and invigorate yang, which tonifies the essential substances, blood and kidney-yang when it is used together with Colla Cornu Cervi. Fructus Psoraleae acts with Colla Cornu Cervi to invigorate kidney and strengthen yang. Semen Biotae used together with Poria serves to keep heart-fire and kidney-water in balance, and tranquilize the patient. Fructus Psoraleae enhances the emission-relieving effect of Cornu Cervi.

Baolong Pill
(Baolong Wan)

Ingredients

Concretio Silicae Bambusae	30 g
Realgar	3 g
Cinnabaris	15 g
Moschus	15 g
Rhizoma Arisaema cum Bile	120 g

Process Grind the above ingredients into powder to make pills.

Efficacy

Clearing away heat, dispersing phlegm, relieving convulsion and fainting; mainly for infants with convulsive seizures attributive to accumulation of phlegm-heat, which manifest as fever, somnolence or loss of consciousness, rough breathing, convulsion, red tongue with yellow, turbid and greasy fur.

Indications

1. Because the prescription contains Realgar and Moschus, it should not be boiled and prepared as decoction.
2. Applicable to infants with convulsion resulting from high fever, accompanied with red tongue and yellow fur, wiry and smooth pulse.
3. Also indicated for cases with epileptic seizures accompanied with yellow, turbid and greasy fur on the tongue, which are attributive to blockage of the orifices by phlegm-heat.
4. Also applicable to cases of uremic coma, hepatic coma and hysteria attributive to accumulation of phlegm-heat; and to cases of encephalitis B, epidemic meningitis, thermoplegia and cerebral malaria marked by high fever and convulsion, which are attributive to attack of severe heat and wind.

Interpretation

Concretio Silicae Bambusae has the effects of clearing away heat, eliminating phlegm, cooling heart-fire and relieving convulsion. Arisaema cum Bile can disperse phlegm, suppress wind and relieve convulsion. The combination of two serves as the principal drugs for the treatment of convulsion of phlegm-heat type. Realgar can eliminate phlegm and toxic material. Moschus is used for waking up the patient from unconsciousness, and Cinnabaris for tranquilizing. The last three drugs together exert a strong anti-convulsive and resuscitating effect.

Bolus for Activating Meridians
(Huo Luo Dan)

Ingredients

Radix Aconiti Praeparata	6 g
Radix Aconiti Kusnezoffii Praeparata	6 g
Lumbricus	10 g

Rhizoma Arisaema cum Bile Praeparata	10 g
Olibanum	3 g
Myrrha	3 g

Efficacy

Warming the channels, activating the circulation of collaterals, expelling wind evil, eliminating dampness and phlegm and removing blood stasis; mainly for cases with prolonged numbness and pain of the extremities, atttributive to retention of wind-phlegm and blood stasis in the meridians.

Indications

1. Applicable to cases of arthralgia of wind- cold-dampness type manifested as prolonged immobility and pain of joints, numbness of muscles and skin, white and greasy fur on the tongue, wiry and smooth pulse.

2. Also applicable to cases of stroke attributive to obstruction of meridians by wind-phlegm, which are manifested as hemiplegia, spasm of limbs, white and greasy fur on the tongue and wiry pulse.

3. Also applicable to cases of Guillain-Barre syndromes, plexus brachialis neuralgia, ischialgia, multiple neuritis, etc., marked by pain of limbs, which are attributive to obstruction of meridians by wind-phlegm and blood stasis, or cases of reheumatic arthritis and cerebral accidents, which are attributive to attack of wind-cold-dampness or obstruction of the meridians by wind-phlegm.

Interpretation

Radix Aconiti Praeparata and Radix Aconiti Kusnezoffii Praeparata can warm the channels, activate the circulation of collaterals and elimintae cold dampness evil from the meridians, and also expel wind evil and relieve pain. Rhizoma Arisaema cum Bile Praeparata can expel wind-phlegm from the meridians, relieve spasm and pain. The above three drugs constituent an effective remedy for eliminating wind-phlegm and blood stasis from meridians. Olibanum and Myrrha serve to disperse blood stasis from the meridians, and the wine can enhance their effects. Lumbricus is helpful to dredge and activate the meridians. In sum, the prescription aims at eliminating wind-phlegm and blood stasis from the meridians, and then relieving pain.

Bolus for Severe Endogenous Wind-Syndrome
(Da Ding Feng Zhu)

Ingredients

Radix Paeoniae Alba	18 g
Radix Rehmanniae	18 g
Colla Corii Asini	10 g
Radix Ophiopogonis	10 g
Plastrum Testudinis	12 g
Concha Ostreae	12 g
Carapax Trionycis	12 g
Semen Sesami	6 g
Fructus Schisandrae	6 g
Radix Glycyrrhizae Praeparata	3 g
Fresh egg yolk	1

Efficacy

Nourishing yin and calming wind, mainly for cases of clonic convulsion attributive to damge of true-yin by heat and hyperactivity of liver-wind, which are accompanied with listlessness, crimson and uncoated tongue, small and weak pulse.

Indications

1. Indicated for cases attributive to deficiency of liver-yin and kidney-yin and upward attack of liver-yang, which are manifested as dizziness aggravated by over

strain or anger, soreness of the loin and knees, insomnia and dreaminess, nocturnal emission, fatigue, bright red tongue, small and rapid pulse.

2. Also applicable to cases of encephalitis B, epidemic meningitis, poliomyelitis and chorea, marked by convulsion, which are attributive to damage of true-yin by heat and hyperactivity of liver-wind.

Interpretation

Egg yolk and Colla Corii Asini are applied to nourish yin-fluid, supplement the exhausted true-yin and calm liver-wind. Rehmanniae, Sesami, Ophiopogonis and Paeoniae Alba serve to nourish yin and blood, soothe the liver and calm wind. Plastrum Testudinis, Concha Ostreae and Carapax Trionycis can invigorate kidney-yin and suppress hyperactive liver-yang.

Radix Glycyrrhizae Praeparata and Fructus Schisandrae are helpful for yin nourishing and wind calming.

Bolus of Arisaematis
(Tiannanxing Wan)

Ingredients

Arisaema cum Bile	10 g
Radix Angelicae Dahuriacae	10 g
Radix Ledebouriellae	10 g
Rhizoma et Radix Notopterygii	10 g
Radix Angelicae Pubescentis	10 g
Rhizoma Ligustici Chuanxiong	10 g
Rhizoma Gastrodiae 10 g	
Radix Paeoniae Alba	10 g
Bombyx Batryticatus	10 g
Herba Ephedrae	6 g
Radix Platycodi	6 g
Herba Asari	6 g

Radix Glycyrrhizae Praeparata	6 g
Rhizoma Zingiberis	6 g
Borneolum Syntheticum	3 g
Moschus	0.6 g

Process All the above ingredients are to be prepared with honey as boluses.

Efficacy

Expelling wind evil and phlegm, waking up the patient and dredging the meridians; mainly for cases of stroke attributed to accumulation of wind-phlegm evil in the interior, which are manifested as numbness of limbs, hemiplegia, aphasia, whitish and greasy fur on the tongue, floating and smooth pulse.

Indications

1. Applicable to cases with swelling pain and immobility of joints, numbness of skin and muscle, whitish and greasy fur on the tongue, smooth pulse, which are attributed to artharalgia of wind-cold-dampness type.

2. Also applicable to cases of cerebral accidents, chronic rheumatic arthritis, sciatica, cervical vertebra syndrome, etc. manifested as hemiplegia, or arthralgia, or numbness of limbs, which are attributed to accumulation of wind-phlegm evil in the interior or arthralgia of wind-cold-dampness type.

Interpretation

Arisaema cum Bile has a potent effect of expelling wind-phlegm evil and dredging the meridians, and acts as the chief drugs in the prescription. Bombyx Batryticatus enhances the effect of Arisaema cum Bile; Ledebouriellae, Notopterygii, Angelicae Pubescentis, Angelicae Dahuricae and Herba Menthae are helpful to expel wind evil and eliminate the dampness evil. Since phlegm-dampness evil is of yin nature, so Zingiberis and Asari are applied to warm the meridians and expel cold evil, and also help Arisaema cum Bile to dry the dampness and eliminate phlegm, so that the mobility of the extremities will be restored. Borneolum Syntheticum and Moschus have the effect of dredging the meridians, and are helpful to relieve aphasia. Gastrodiae, Glycyrrhizae Praeparata, Ligustici Chuanxiong and Paeoniae Alba have the effects of regulating vital energy and blood, subduing endogenous wind evil and relieving convulsion.

Bolus of Placenta Hominis
(Heche Ba Wei Wan)

Ingredients

Placenta Hominis 1 *set* (*cooked with ginger juice and wine*)	
Fructus Corni	30 g
Radix Ophiopogonis	30 g
Radix Rehmanniae Praeparata	90 g
(*cooked with ginger juice and Fructus Amomi*)	
Cortex Moutan Radicis	15 g
Rhizoma Alismatis	15 g
Cornu Cervi Pantotrichum	60 g
Fructus Schisandrae	60 g
Rhizoma Dioscoreae	165 g
Poria	45 g
Radix Aconiti Praeparata	22 g
Ramulus Cinnamomi	22 g

Process   Grind the above ingredients into powder to make pills with honey.

Efficacy

Invigorating kidney, benefiting essence and vital energy and nourishing blood; mainly for cases attributive to impairment of kidney-energy and insufficiency of lung and spleen qi after epileptic seizures, which manifest as spiritlessness, dizziness, palpitation, lumbago, fatigue of the lower limbs, aversion to cold, weakness, poor appetite, loose stools, pale and corpulent tongue with white and smooth fur, slow and weak pulse.

Indications

1. Indicated for infantile maldevelopment manifested by tardiness of ability to walk, delayed growth of the teeth, weakness of the tendon and bone, pale tongue with white fur, sunken and weak pulse, which are attributive to insufficiency of kidney-yang.
2. Also for cases of sterility, impotence or nocturnal emission accompanied with dizziness, tinnitus, lumbago, cold limbs, pale and corpulent tongue with white and smooth fur, which are attributive to the impairment of kidney-yang and insufficiency of essence and blood.
3. Applicable to cases of leukorrhagia with profuse thin discharge, lumbago, fatigue, feeling of coldness over the lower abdomen, nocturia, spiritlessness, which are attributive to the weakness of kidney qi and loss of essence fluid.
4. Also applicable to cases of senile dementia and climacterium syndrome with spiritlessness, which are attributive to the impairment of kidney qi and insufficiency of lung and spleen qi; and to cases of endometritis and senile vaginitis with leukorrhagia, which are attributive to weakness of kidney qi and loss of essence substance.

Interpretation

The prescription is formed by adding Placenta Hominis, Ophiopogonis, Cornu Cervi Pantotrichum and Schisandrae to Pill for Invigorating Kidney Qi which has the effects of invigorating kidney yin, nourishing liver blood, benefiting spleen yin and strengthening kidney yang. Ophiopogonis and Schisandrae used together with the Boluses serves to nourish the lung and kidney. Cornu Cervi Pantotrichum is used for promoting the production of essence and marrow and benefiting qi. Placenta Hominis has a strong effect of tonifying qi and blood, and is available for various kinds of consumptive diseases.

Bolus of Precious Drugs
(Zhi Bao Dan)

Ingredients

Cornu Rhinocerotis	30 g
Carapax Eretmochelydis	30 g
Succinum	30 g
Cinnabaris	30 g
Realgar	30 g
Borneolum Syntheticum	0.3 g
Moschus	0.3 g
Calculus Bovis	15 g
Benzoinum	45 g
Gold sheet	50 pcs (half for coating)
Silver sheet	50 pcs

Process All the above drugs are ground into powder and prepared into boluses, each weighs 3 g.

Efficacy

Eliminating dampness-phlegm, waking up patients from unconsciousness, clearing away heart-fire and detoxifying; mainly for cases of coma, profuse expectoration, heavy breath, fever, restlessness, red tongue with yellowish, greasy and dirty fur, smooth and rapid pulse, which are attributive to the attack of the interior by heat evil and stagnation of dampness-phlegm, also for the infantile convulsion due to stagnation of phlegm-heat.

Indications

1. Applicable to cases of sudden fainting or apoplexy attributive to the attack of percardium by phlegm-heat although there is no fever.

2. Applicable to cases of sunstroke attributive to stagnation of dampness-phlegm and retention of summer-heat.

3. It has been recorded in Prescription of People's Welfare Pharmacy that the bolus is taken with ginger juice to enhance the effect of waking up a patient.

4. Also applicable to comatose cases of hepatic coma, cerebrovascular accident, epilepsy, uremia, etc. which are attributive to retention of heat and dampness-phlegm.

Interpretation

Calculus Bovis can eliminate phlegm, wake up one from unconciousness, clear away heart-fire and has the effect of detoxication. Its action is strong and rapid, so it is used as the principal drug. Moschu, Borneolum Syntheticum and Benzoinum have the effects of exorcising evils, dissipating dampness-phlegm and restoring consciousness; Cornu Rhinocerotis and Carapax Eretmochelydis can clear away heart-fire and have the action of detoxication. Realgar has the effect of detoxication and Cinnabaris, Succinum, gold sheet and silver sheet have the effect of tranquilizing. The combination of these drugs constitutes a prescription with eliminating dampness-phlegm and waking up one from unconsciousness as the chief effect, and with clearing away heart-fire and detoxifying as the auxiliary one. This is different from Bolus of Calculus Bovis for Resurrection.

Bolus of Storax
(Suhexiang Wan)

Ingredients

Rhizoma Atractylodis Macrocephalae	60 g
Radix Aucklandiae	60 g
Cornu Rhinocerotis	60 g
Rhizoma Cyperi	60 g
Cinnabaris	60 g
Fructus Chebulae	60 g
Lignum Santali	60 g
Benzoinum	60 g

Lignum Aquilariae Resinatum	60 g
Moschus	60 g
Flos Caryophylli	60 g
Fructus Piperis Longi	60 g
Borneolum Syntheticum	30 g
Oleum Storax	30 g
Olibanumm	30 g

Process   *All the above ingredients are prepared with honey to make boluses.*

Efficacy

Warming and dredging the meridians to wake up patients from unconsciousness. sciousness, promoting the circulation of vital energy and eliminating the dampness evil; mainly for cases due to the obstruction of vital energy circulation by Relieve cold or phlegm- dampness evil and impairment of consciousness, which are manifested as sudden syncope, lockjaw, cyanosis and pallor, cold breath, whitish and smooth fur on the tongue, sunken, slow and strong pulse.

Indications

1. Applicable to cases of angina pectoris attributive to stagnation of cold evil and vital energy or attack of dampness evil.

2. May be used as an emergency treatment for cases due to phlegm obstruction of the heart, manifested as epileptic seizures, mental upset, staring eyes, paraphasia, whitish and greasy fur on the tongue, before other causative treatments are applied.

3. Indicated only for cold type asthenia- syndrome of coma.

4. Also applicable to comatose cases of cerebral accidents, uremia, hepatic coma, etc.; mental disorders occuring in psychosis, such as schizophrenia, symptomatic psychosis, etc.; chest pain occuring in angina pectoris and myocardial infarction; which are attributive to the obstruction of vital energy circulation by cold or phlegm-dampness evil.

Interpretation

This prescription is a typical preescription for waking up patient from unconsciousness, which composed of many aromatic drugs such as Storax, Benzoinum, Moschus and Borneolum Syntheticum, Cornu Rhinocerotis has the effects of clearing away heart-fire and eliminating toxic material; Cinnabaris, that of tranquilizing. The above six drugs used together are effective for waking up the patient from unconsciousness and for tranquilizing. Santali, Caryophylli, Cyperi, Aquilariae Resinatum, Pipers Longi, Boswelliae Olibanum and Atractylodis Macrocephalae constitute another group of herbs for regulating the function of viscera and enhancing the dampness-dispersing and waking effect. Chebulae of warm and astringing nature is added to prevent the damage of healthy energy by the aromatic drugs.

Brain-Invigorating and Kidney-Tonifying Pill
(Jian Nao Bu Shen Wan)

Ingredients

Semen Ziziphi Spinosae
Radix Polygalae
Os Draconis Fossilia Ossis Mastodi
Radix Cyathulae
Cortex Eucommiae
Cinnabaris
Radix Angelicae Sinensis
Rhizoma Dioscoreae
Radix Ginseng
Cornu Cervi Pantotrichum

Efficacy

Invigorating the brain, replenishing qi, tonifying the kidney and strengthening the essence of life.

Indications

Applicable to cases of neurosis, amnesia, insomnia, dizziness, vertigo, tinnitus, palpitation, lassitude in loin and knees, emission due to kidney deficiency, etc..

Cardiotonic Pill
(Tianwang Buxin Dan)

Ingredients

Radix Rehmanniae	120 g
Radix Scrophulariae	60 g
Radix Salviae Miltiorrhizae	60 g
Radix Angelicae Sinensis	60 g
Radix Ginseng	60 g
Poria	60 g
Semen Biotae	60 g
Semen Ziziphi Spinosae	60 g
Radix Polygalae	60 g
Radix Asparagi	60 g
Radix Ophiopogonis	60 g
Fructus Schisandrae	60 g
Radix Platycodi	60 g

Directions

Take 9 grams three times daily. It can also be made into decoction, with the dosage modified proportionally according to the original recipe.

Efficacy

Nourishing yin to remove heat and tonifying blood to tranquilize the mind.

Indications

1. Asthenic fire stirring up inside due to deficiency of yin and blood brought on by the hypofunction of heart and kidney marked by insomnia with vexation, palpitation, mental weariness, nocturnal emission, amnesia, dry stools, orolingual boil, reddened tongue with little fur, thready and rapid pulse.
2. Neurosism, paroxysmal tachycardia, hypertension, hyperthyroidism and others marked by the above-mentioned symptoms can be treated by the modified recipe.
3. Modern researches have proved that the recipe has a better effect of regulating the cerebral cortex. It can tranquilize the mind to induce sleep without causing listlessness and achieve the effects of enriching the blood and relieving the symptoms of coronary heart disease.

CAUTIONS

The recipe is composed of nourishing, greasy drugs which affect the stomach, so it is not fit to take for a long time.

Decoction for Activating Blood Circulation
(Tong Qiao Huo Xue Tang)

Ingredients

Radix Paeoniae Rubra	10 g
Rhizoma Ligustici Chuanxiong	10 g
Semen Persicae	10 g

Bulbus Allii Fistulosi   10 g
Rhizoma Zingiberis Recens   10 g
Flos Carthami   6 g
Fructus Ziziphi Jujubae   6 pcs
Moschus   0.3 g
wine q.s.

Efficacy

Activating blood circulation and opening the orificies; mainly for cases of headache and dizziness due to accumulation of blood stasis in the head.

Indications

1. Indicated for cases of alopecia, deafness and sinusitis, which are attributive to accumulation of blood stasis in the head.
2. For cases of sudden loss of vision which are attributive to accumulation of blood stasis in the eyes, omit wine and Ziziphi Jujubae and add Faeces Vespertilionis and Radix Salviae Miltiorrhizae to nourish blood and promote vision.
3. Also applicable to sequelae of cerebral concussion, cases of cerebral arteriosclerosis and cerebellar bleeding with headache and dizziness, and to cases of retinal hemorrhage and embolism of central retinal artery with sudden loss of vision which are attributive to the same mechanism.

Interpretation

Persicae, Carthami, Paeoniae Rubra and Ligustici Chuanxiong have the effects of activating blood circulation and removing blood stasis. Allii Fistulosi and Zingiberis help the above drugs distributing to the vertex. Moschus, fragrant and active, can dredge the passage of meridians and open the orifice, and is particularly suitable for the treatment of headache and dizziness due to accumulation of blood stasis in the head when used together with Persicae and Carthami. Wine and Ziziphi Jujubae used together have the effects of promoting blood flow and distributing the above drugs to the head.

Decoction for Eliminating Dampness and Relieving Rheumatism (Chu Shi Juan Bi Tang)

Ingredients

Rhizoma Atractylodis	12 g
Rhizoma Atractylodis Macrocephalae	10 g
Poria	10 g
Rhizoma seu Radix Notopterygii	10 g
Rhizoma Alismatis	10 g
Exocarpium Citri Grandis	6 g
Radix Glycyrrhizae	3 g
Succus Zingiberis	3 spoonfuls
Succus Bambusae	3 spoonfuls

Efficacy

Strengthening the spleen, eliminating dampness, expelling wind, dissipating phlegm, relieving rheumatism and alleviating pain; mainly for cases of rheumatism manifested as localized arthralgia which will be aggravated in rainy days, fatigue, white and greasy fur on the tongue, wiry and smooth pulse, which are attributive to retention of dampness in the spleen and stomach and attack of wind-phlegm to the meridians and joints.

Indications

1. For cases of apoplexy manifested by distortion of the face, dysphasia, numbness and spasms of limbs, or even ehmiplegia, white and greasy fur on the tongue, wiry and smooth pulse, which are attributive to the attack of meridians by phlegm-dampness, omit Glycyrrhizae and add Scorpio, Bombyx Batryticatus.

2. For cases attributive to the attack of upper orifices by phlegm-dampness, which manifest as vertigo accompanied with nausea, vomiting, tinnitus, deafness, white and greasy tongue fur and wiry pulse, add Rhizoma Pinelliae

Praeparata, Rhizoma Gastrodiae and omit Glycyrrhizae.

3. Also applicable to cases with rheumatic arthritis, sciatica and beriberi attributive to accumulation of dmapness in the spleen and stomach; to cases of facial paralysis, poliomyelitis and thromboangiitis obliterans of cerebral bessels with hemiplesia attributive to attack of meridians by wind-phlegm; and to cases of hypertension and cerebral arteriosclerosis, with dizziness attributive to attack of the upper orifices by phlegm-dampness.

Interpretation

Atractylodis acts as the chief drug in the prescription and is applied in large dosage, which has the effects of activating the spleen, drying dampness, eliminating wind and alleviating pain. Atractylodis Macrocephalae and Poria serve to strengthen the spleen and promote diuresis. Citri Grandis can regulate vital energy and acitivate the spleen, thus assists in eliminating dampness. Succus Zingiberis and Lophatheri are used to expel wind, dredge meridians and dissipate phlegm.

Decoction for Hemiplegia
(Xu Ming Tang)

Ingredients

Lignum Cinnamomi	9 g
Radix Paeoniae Alba	9 g
Rhizoma Zingiberis	6 g
Herba Ephedrae	6 g
Rhizoma Ligustici Chuanxiong	6 g
Radix Codonopsis Pilosulae	6 g
Semen Armeniacae Amarum	6 g
Radix Angelicae Sinensis	9 g
Gypsum Fibrosum	15 g
Radix Glycyrrhizae	3 g

Efficacy

Warming meridians, nourishing blood and expelling wind.

Indications

It is indicated for cases of hemiplegia after apoplexy, accompanied with weakness and rigidity of limbs, pale tongue with whitish fur, wiry and small pulse. Nowadays, it is usually applied for sequela of stroke. The action of this prescription is similar as that of the former, but its effect of warming meridians and strengthening yang energy is milder and has an additional effect of nourishing blood and expelling wind. It is suitable for cases of stroke attributive to deficiency of vital energy and blood and attack of the meridians by wind.

Decoction for Invigorating Spleen and Nourishing heart (Gui Pi Tang)

Ingredients

Radix Astragali seu Hedysari	15 g
Radix Codonopsis Pilosulae	15 g
Radix Angelicae Sinensis	12 g
Arillus Longan	12 g
Rhizoma Atractylodis Macrocephalae	10 g
Poria	10 g
Semen Ziziphi Spinosae	10 g
Radix Aucklandiae	5 g
Radix Glycyrrhizae Praeparata	5 g
Radix Polygalae	3 g
Rhizoma Zingiberis Recens	5 pcs
Fructus Ziziphi Jujubae	5 pcs

Indications

Benefiting vital energy, strengthening spleen, invigorating the heart and nourishing blood; mainly for cases due to hypofunction of heart and spleen and insufficiency of vital energy and blood, manifested as palpitation, amnesia, insomnia, fatigue poor appetite, sallow complexion, or preceded menstrual cycle with profuse pale or continuously dripping discharge, pale tongue with whitish fur, small and weak pulse. For cases of metrorrhagia attributive to failure of the spleen to control blood, subtract Aucklandiae and polygalae and add Fructus Corni to nourish liver and stop metrorrhagia. For case with hematochezia attributive to hypofunction of spleen with retention of cold evil, subtract Polygalae and add Zingiberis Praeparata to warm middle jiao and stopping bleeding. Also applicable to cases of pepticulcer, dysfunctional uterine bleeding, thrombocytopenia purpura, aplastic anemia etc. with hemorrhage attributive to hypofunction of heart and spleen.

Interpretation

Astragali seu Hedysari and Codonopsis Pilosulae benefit vital energy and invigorate the spleen and serve as the chief drugs. Angelicae Sinensis and Arillus Longan tonify the blood, nourish the heart. The above four drugs used together strengthen both the heart and the spleen, and dealt with the primary aspect of the disease. Poria, Polygalae, Ziziphi Spinosae have the effects of nourishing the heart and calming the mental state, and dealt with the secondary aspect of the disease. Aucklandiae adn Atractylodis Macrocephalae strengthen the spleen adn regulate vital energy. Glycyrrhizae, Zingiberis Recens and Ziziphi Jujubae reconcile the action of spleen and stomach and promote the production of vital energy and blood. In summary, this prescription aims at benefiting vital energy and tonifying blood, when one's vital energy is sufficient, the heart is well nourished, the symptoms subside.

Decoction for Invigorating Yang
(Bu Yang Huan Wu Tang)

Ingredients

Radix Astragali seu Hedysari	60 g
Radix Angelicae Sinensis	15 g
Radix Paeoniae Rubra	15 g
Lumbricus	10 g
Rhizoma Ligustici Chuanxiong	10 g
Semen Persicae	6 g
Flos Carthami	6 g

Efficacy

tonifying vital energy, promoting blood circulation and dredging the meridian passage; mainly for stroke sequelae such as hemiplegia, facial deviation, aphasia, slobbering, lower limbs paralyses, incontinence of urine, etc. with white fur and slow pulse.

Indications

1. For cases of unconsciousness attributed to sthenia-syndrome, the therapy for waking up from unconsciousness should be applied before the prescription is given.

2. The purpose of using crude sample of Astragali seu Hedysari is to remove blood stasis, therefore, a large dosage (beginning from 30-60 g should be applied in order to let it distributing all over the whole body.

3. For cases with much phlegm, add Rhizoma Arisaemacum Bile and Concretio Silicae Bambusae to eliminate the wind-phlegm; while for cases of aphasia, add Rhizoma Acori Graminei and Radix Polygalae to wake up the patient adn eliminate phlegm.

4. For cases of bi-syndrome due to deficiency of vital energy and blood sta-

sis, add Ramulus Taxilli to nourish the blood and eliminate wind evil.

5. The prescription may also be applicable to hemiplegia paraplegia, monoplegia resulting from cerebrovascular accidents and infantile paralysis, and rheumatic arthritis, rheumatoid arthritis, etc. attributed to deficiency of vital energy and blood stasis.

Interpretation

Astragali seu Hedysari is the principal drug in this prescription, while has the effect of tonifying vital energy to promote blood circulation. The other ingredients have the effects of promoting blood circulation and dredging the meridiean passage. The prescription, as a whole, can tonify vital energy and also promote blood circulation, remove blood stasis but not hurt the healthy energy. When the vital energy is sufficient, the blood flow activated, the blood stasis is removed and the meridian passage is dredged, all the above-metioned disorders will be relieved.

Decoction for Mild Hemiplegia
(Xiao Xu Ming Tang)

Ingredients

Lignum Cinnamomi	9 g
Radix Aconiti Praeparata	9 g
Radix Paeoniae Alba	9 g
Radix Ledebouriellae	9 g
Rhizoma zingiberis Recens	9 g
Herba Ephedrae	6 g
Rhizoma Ligustici Chuanxiong	6 g
Radix Codonopsis Pilosulae	6 g
Semen Armeniacae Amarum	6 g
Radix Scutellariae	6 g
Radix Stephaniae Tetrandrae	6 g

Radix Glycyrrhizae   3 g

Efficacy

Warming meridians, promoting the motion of yang- energy, supporting healthy energy and eliminating wind; mainly for cases of hemiplegia accompanied with distortion of the face, aphasia, spasm of limbs, headache, rigid neck, whitish fur on the tongue, tense pulse, which are attributive to deficiency of healthy energy and attack of wind-cold to meridians.

Indications

1. Applicable to rheumatism of wind-cold- dampness type with insufficiency of yang-energy, which manifests as wandering arthralgia, numbness of muscles and skin, limited movement of joints, white and smooth fur on the tongue, wiry and tense pulse.

2. This prescription is only suitable for stroke due to attack of the meridians by exogenous wind but contraindicated for cases of hemiplegia with distortion of the face of loss of consciousness which are attributive to impairment of liver and kidney, and the attack of asthenic wind inside the body.

3. Also applicable to cases of cerebral thrombosis and periodic paralysis with hemiplegia attributive to attack of meridians by wind-cold and to cases of chronic gouty arthritis, rheumatoid spondylitis, hyperplastic arthritis, etc. with arthralgia attributive to insufficiency of yang-energy and the attack of exogenous wind-cold-dampness.

Interpretation

Ephedrae, ledebouriellae, Ligustic Chuanxiong and Armeniacae Amarum have the effects of dispelling superficial evils and warming and dredging meridians. Cinnamomi, Paeoniae Alba, Zingiberis Recens and Glycyrrhizae can regulate ying and wei, and not only enhance the effects of the above drugs but also increase the body resistance to defend against the attack of wind. Codonopsis Pilosulae and Aconiti Praeparata are used for benefiting vital energy and blood to restore the healthy energy and eliminate the evils when used with Paeoniae Alba and Ligustici Chuanxiong. Stephaniae Tetrandrae and Scutellariae can clear away the superficial heat and expel wind. Originally, there was Lignum Cinnamomi in the prescription, but it was often replaced by Ramulus Cinnamomi in the clinic. The former is good for warming the kidney to support yang, while the latter is for expelling wind, promoting sweating and warming and dredging the meridians. They may be applied accordingly.

Decoction for Removing Blood Stasis in the Chest (Xue Fu Zhu Yu Tang)

Ingredients

Radix Angelicae Sinensis	9 g
Rhizoma Ligustici Chuanxiong	5 g
Radix Paeoniae Rubra	9 g
Semen Persicae	12 g
Flos Carthami	9 g
Radix Bupleuri	3 g
Radix Platycodi	5 g
Fructus Aurantii	6 g
Radix Rehmanniae	9 g
Radix Glycyrrhizae	3 g
Radix Achyranthis Bidentatae	9 g

All the above drugs are to be decocted in water for oral administration.

Efficacy

Promoting blood circulation to remove blood stasis and promoting circulation of qi to relieve pain.

Indications

1. Syndrome of blood stasis in the chest marked by long-standing prickly chest pain and headache which exist in a certain region, or endless hiccup, dysphoria due to interior heat, palpitation, insomnia, irritability and liability to a fit of temper, running a fever gradually at dusk, deep-red tongue with ecchymoses, dark-purple lips or dark eyes, uneven pulse or taut and tense pulse. Coronary heart disease, cerebral thrombosis, thromboangiitis, obliterans, hypertension, cirrhosis of liver, dysmenorrhea, amenia, headache, chest pain and hypochondriac pain marked by stagnancy of qi and blood stasis can be treated by the modified recipe.

Interpretation

The leading ingredients in the recipe are Radix Angelicae Sinensis, Rhizoma Ligustici Chuanxiong, Radix Paeoniae Rubra, Semen Persicae, Flos Carthami and Radix Bupleuri, which promote blood circulation to remove blood stasis. Among them, Radix Bupleuri also ensures proper downward flow of the blood. Radix Platycodi soothes the liver and regulates the circulation of qi. Fructus Aurantii and Radix Rehmanniae relieve the oppressed feeling in the chest, promote the circulation of qi to render blood circulation to be normal. Radix Achyranthis Bidentatae removes heat from the blood and combines Radix Angelicae Sinensis to enrich the blood and moisten dryness so as to remove blood stasis without impairment of yin. Radix Glycyrrhizae cooridinates the effects of all the other ingredients in the recipe. Modern researches have proved that this recipe is especially effective in anti-coagulation and antispasm. Besides, it has some effect on uterine contraction.

CAUTIONS

1. Since this recipe is mainly composed of drugs for removing blood stasis, it should not be used to treat the syndrome without distinct stasis.
2. Contraindicated for pregnant cases.

Decoction for Sterility
(Hua Shui Zhong Zi Tang)

Ingredients

Radix Morindae Officinalis (soaked in salt solution)	10 g
Poria	10 g
Radix Codonopsis Pilosulae	10 g
Semen Cuscutae (fried with wine)	10 g
Semen Euryales (fried)	10 g
Rhizoma Atractylodis Macrocephalae (fried with earth)	12 g
Semen Plantaginis (fried with wine)	6 g
Cortex Cinnamomi	2 g

Efficacy

Warming the kidney, strengthening the spleen and promoting diuresis, mainly for cases of sterility accompanied with lumbago, aversion to cold, cold limbs, fatigue, flat taste in the mouth, poor appetite, oliguria, edema of the lower limbs, puffiness of the body, corpulent tongue with white and greasy fur, sunken and slow pulse, which are attributive to deficiency of spleen-yang and kidney-yang, and retention of dampness in the uterus.

Indications

1. Applicable to cases of impotence or nocturnal emission accompanied with dizziness, spiritlessness, lumbago, weakness of lower limbs, pale complexion, poor appetite, loose stools, pale tongue with white fur, sunken and slow pulse, which are attributive to declination of life-gate fire and deficiency of kidney-qi.

2. Also indicated for cases with general pitted edema which is more prominent in the lower part, lumbago, fatigue, cold limbs, aversion to cold, oliguria, poor appetite, loose stools, corpulent tongue with white smooth fur, sunken and

slow pulse, which are attributive to deficiency of spleen-yang and kidney-yang and accumulation of cold-dampness in the interior.

3. Also applicable to cases of endocrine disorder such as hypothyroidism, and pelvic diseases such as endometritis with sterility attributive to deficiency of spleen-yang and retention of dampness in the uterus; to cases of hypogonadism and neurasthenia with impotence or nocturnal emission attributive to the declination of life-gate fire and deficiency of kidney-qi; and to cases of chronic nephritis with edema attributive to deficiency of spleen-yang and kidney-yang and accumulation of cold-dampness in the interior.

Decoction for Treating Rheumatism
(Juan Bi Tang)

Ingredients

Rhizoma seu Radix Notopterygii	10 g
Rhizoma Curcumae Longae 10 g	
Radix Angelicae Sinensis (soaked with wine) 10 g	
Radix Paeoniae Alba	10 g
Radix Ledebouriellae	10 g
Radix Astragalae seu hedysari	15 g
Radix Glycyrrhizae Praeparata	6 g
Rhizoma Zingiberis Recens	5 pcs

Efficacy

Expelling wind and dampness, benefiting vital energy and nourishing blood; mainly for rheumatism of wind type attributive to the stagnation of wind-cold-dampness evil (predominantly the wind evil) in the meridians, which is manifested as immobility of the joints, wandering arthralgia, especially the neck, back, shoulder and elbow, thin and white fur on the tongue, floating and slow pulse.

Indications

1. Applicable to cases of stroke manifested by deviation of the eyes and mouth, numbness of the muscles and skin, spasm of limbs, or hemiplegia (especially the upper limb), thin and whitish fur on the tongue, floating and wiry pulse, which are attributive to weakness of the superficies, deficiency of vital energy and attack of wind evil.

2. Also applicable to cases of rheumatic arthritis, rheumtoid arthritis, facial paralysis, cerebral accidents, etc., which are attributive to the stagnation of wind-cold-dampness evil (predominantly the wind evil) in the meridians.

Interpretation

Nontopterygii and Ledebouriellae can expel wind evil, remove dampness evil and relieve pain, and is especially suitable for rheumatism of the upper body. Astragali seu Heday sari and Glycyrrhizae Praeparata have the effects of supp0lementing vital energy and strengthening the body surface and is helpful for expelling wind evil. Meanwhile, Astragali seu Heday sari and Glycyrrhizae Praeparata exert a tonifying effect without causing indigestion, and Notopterygii and Ledebouriellae promote vital energy circulation without losing it when all are used together. Angelicae Sinensis and Paeoniae Alba can nourish blood and promote blood circulation, Curcumae Longae is used for regulating vital energy in the blood; they are applied together for nourishing the blood to eliminate wind. Zingiberis Recens helps Notopterygii and Ledebouriellae to expel wind and dampness, and also helps Astragali seu Hedysari and Glycyrrhizae Praeparata to cooridinate ying-qi and wei-qi. Therefore, the prescription is also suitable for bi-syndrome due to wind-cold-dampness evil, characterized by deficiency of both ying-qi and wei-qi.

Decoction of Bupleuri Adding Os Draconis and Concha Ostreae
(Chaihu Jia Longgu Muli Tang)

Ingredients

Radix Bupleuri	10 g
Radix Sutellariae	6 g
Rhizoma zingiberis Recens	6 g
Radix Codonopsis Pilosulae	6 g
Ramulus Cinnamomi	6 g
Radix et Rhizoma Rhei	6 g
Poria	6 g
Rhizoma Pinelliae	6 g
Minium	1 g
Fructus Ziziphi Jujubae	3 pcs
Os Draconis	15 g
Concha Ostreae	15 g

Efficacy

Regulating shaoyang, dispersing phlegm, tranquilizing, supporting healthy energy and eliminating evil; mainly for cases attributive to invasion of heat to shaoyang (liver and gallbladder), which manifest feeling of oppression over the chest and hypochondrium, restlessness, delirium, frightening, insomnia, fatigue, red tongue with yellow fur, wiry and rapid pulse, i.e., the simultaneous occurence of asthenia- and sthenia-syndrome, cold= and heat-syndrome, as well as superficies- and interior-syndrome.

Indications

1. Minium is a poinsonous drug and should not be taken more than 10 g at one time and not for a long period. Now it is usually replaced by Ferrum scale.
2. Applicable to cases of epilepsy accom= panied with dizziness, fatigue,

pale complexion, red tongue with white and greasy fur, wiry and smooth pulse, which are attributive to adverse rising of wind-phlegm with simultaneous occurence of asthenia- and sthenia-syndrome.

3. Also indicated for cases of tinnitus and deafness accompanied with profuse expectoration, bitter taste in the mouth, feeling of oppression over the chest and hypochondrium, dizziness, fatigue, red tongue with yellow fur, wiry and rapid pulse, which are attributive to the adverse rising of phlegm-fire from the liver and gallbladder, with simultaneous occurence of asthenia- and sthenia-syndrome.

4. Also applicable to cases of hyperthyroidism, schizophrenia and neurasthenia marked by palpitation, which are attributive to the invasion of heat to shaoyang (liver and gallbladder); and to cases of Meniere's syndrome and sequelae of cerebral concussion marked by tinnitus and dizziness, which are attributive to adverse rising of phlegm- fire from the liver, gallbladder, with simultaneous occurrence of asthenia- and sthenia-syndrome.

Interpretation

The prescription is composed on the basis of the Decoction of Bupleuri for Regulating Shaoyang , by adding Ramulus Cinnamomi, Rhei, Poria, Minium, Os Draconis, Concha Ostreae and omitting Glycyrrhizae from it. Bupleuri serves to eliminate the pathogens from the interior when it is used together with Ramulus Cinnamomi and to clear away the heat located between the superificies and the interior when it is used together with Scutellariae. Rhei can directly clear away the interior heat. Pinelliae, Zingiberis Recens and Minium disperse phlegm and eliminate accumulated heat. Os Draconis and Concha Ostreae act as sedative. Codonopsis Pilosulae, Ziziphi Jujubae and Poria are applied for strengthening the spleen, benefiting vital energy and supporting healthy energy. In sum, the prescription aims at eliminating pathogens both from the superficies and interior by applying drugs both cold and warm in ntaure, tonifying and purging as well as descending and ascending in action.

Decoction of Bupleuri and Puerariae for Expelling Evil from Musices
(Chai Ge Jie Ji Tang)

Ingredients

Radix Bupleuri	10 g
Radix Puerariae	10 g
Gypsum Fibrosum	10 g
Radix Scutellariae	6 g
Radix Paeoniae Lactiflorae	6 g
Rhizoma seu Radix Notopterygii	6 g
Radix Angelicae Dahuriae	6 g
Radix Glycyrrhizae	3 g
Radix Platycodi	3 g
Rhizoma Zingiberis Recens	3 pcs
Fructus Ziziphi Jujubae	3 pcs

Efficacy

Expelling the evil from the superficies, lowering fever and clearing away the interior heat evil; mainly for common cold of wind-cold type with formation of heat, which is manifested by chilliness becoming milder and fever higher, headache, soreness of limbs, eyes pain, thin and yellowish fur on the tongue, floating and bounding pulse, etc..

Indications

1. For cases of warm-type malaria manifested by high fever, mild chilliness, general aching, red tongue with yellowish fur, wiry and rapid pulse, omit Radix Glycyrrhizae and Radix Platycodi and add Fructus Tsaoko eliminate dampness.

2. For cases of heat-type arthralgia manifested by joint aching, fever, chilliness, yellowish and greasy fur on the tongue, omit Radix Glycyrrhizae and Radix Platycodi, and add Cortex Phellodendri and Ramulus Cinnamomi to eliminate dampness-heat, dredge the meridians and relieve pain.

3. Applicable to cases of wind-fire toothache manifested by toothache referring to the head, chilliness, red tongue with whitish fur, wiry pulse.

4. Also applicable to cases of influenza, trigeminal neuralgia, rheumatic arthritis, etc. which are attributive to heat formation by stagnation of cold.

Interpretation

Bupleuri and Puerariae have the effects of expelling the evil from the superficies and lowering fever. Notopterygii and Angelica Dahuricae have the effect of expelling wind evil from the body surface. Scutellariae and Gypsum Fibrosum have the effect of clearing away the interior heat evil. Paeoniae Lactiflorae is helpful to regulate ying and clear away heat evil. Platycodi helps Bupleuri to expel evil. Zingiberis Recens, Ziziphi Jujubae and Glycyrrhizae regulate the function of ying and wei and then the middle jiao. Although this prescription composes of the drugs of cold nature as well as those of warm nature, but, as a whole, its cold nature is greater than warm nature. However, it is still a prescription of acrid flavour and cool nature, which expels wind-heat.

Decoction of Cimicifugae and Astragali seu Hedysari
(Shengma Huangqi Tang)

Ingredients

Radix Astragali seu Hedysari	30 g
Radix Angelicae Sinensis	12 g
Rhizoma Cimicifugae	6 g
Radix Bupleuri	6 g

Efficacy

Benefiting vital energy, lifting yang and activating vital energy; mainly for cases of dysuria attributive to dysfunction of vital energy, which manifest difficult and dripping urination, tiredness, shortness of breath; pale tongue, slow and weak pulse.

Indications

1. For cases attributing to deficiency and collapes of vital energy and downward flowing of essential substance, which manifest prolonged discharge of rice-water like urine, pale complexion, fatigue, pale tongue and feeble pulse, add Fructus Corni to keep the essential substance.

2. for protracted cases of nocturnal emission or enuresis accompanied with listlessness, pale complexion, pale tongue, sunken and feeble pulse, which are attributive to deficiency of vital energy, add Fructus Schisandrae and Ootheca Mantidis to calm the mental state and astringe the essential substance (or urine).

3. Also applicable to cases of chronic prostatitis, neurasthenia, senile dementia, etc. with difficult urination or enuresis, which are attributive to dysfunction of vital energy.

Interpretation

This prescription is developed from the Decoction for Strengthening Middle Jiao and Benefiting Qi which is mainly for collapse of middle-jiao energy and hypofunction of spleen and stomach. In the prescription, Astragalic seu Hedysari is applied together with Cimicifugae for supplementing vital energy and raising yang to restore with Cimicifugae for supplementing vital energy and raising yang to restore the normal function of vital energy. Angelicae Sinensis and Bupleuri can disperse the stagnated liver-energy. In sum, the purpose of this prescription is to lift up collapse vital energy and restore the normal urination.

Decoction of Cinnamomi Aconiti
(Guizhi Fuzi Tang)

Ingredients

Ramulus Cinnamomi	12 g
Radix Aconiti Praeparata	10 g
Rhizoma Zingiberis Recens	10 g
Fructus Ziziphi Jujubae	8 pcs
Radix Glycyrrhizae Praeparata	6 g

Efficacy

Expelling wind and dampness, warming meridians and eliminating cold; mainly for cases attributive to the attack of wind-cold-dampness to the muscles and meridians, and circulatory impediment of vital energy and blood, which manifest general aching, immovability of trunk and limbs, no thirst nor vomiting, white and greasy fur, floating and unsmooth pulse.

Indications

1. Applicable to cases with a yang-deficiency constitution and affection of wind-cold, which manifest chilliness, fever, aversion to wind, sweating, headache, cold limbs, tiredness of somnolence, white and greasy fur, sunken and slow pulse.

2. Also indicated for cases with chest apin referring to the back, feeling of oppression over the chest, tiredness, white and greasy fur on the tongue, wiry and slow pulse, which are attributive to accumulation of cold-dampness.

3. Also applicable to cases of rheumatic arthritis, sciatic periomarthritis, etc. with chillness and fever attributive to yang-deficiency and affection of exogenous wind-cold; and to cases of emphysema, coronary heart disease, rheumatic heart disease, etc. with chest pain attributive to accumulation of wind-phlegm.

Interpretation

Aconiti has the effects of warming the meridians and eliminating cold-dmapness from the meridians. They two act as the principal drugs of the prescription. Zingiberis Recens and Ziziphi Jujubae serve to regulate ying and wei and can warm the meridians and promote the circulation of vital energy and blood when they are used together with Cinnamomi.

Decoction of Cinnamomi, Glycyrrhizae, etc.
(Guizhi Gancao Longgu Muli Tang)

Ingredients

Ramulus Cinnamomi	10 g
Radix Clycyrrhizae Praeparata	15 g
Os Draconis	30 g
Concha Ostreae	30 g

Efficacy

Warming heart-yang energy and tranquilizing; mainly for cases attributive to impairment of heart-yang, which manifest palpitation, irritability, spontaneous sweating, pale tongue with white and greasy fur, floating and slow, or slow pulse with irregular intervals.

Indications

1. For cases attributive to severe deficiency of heart-yang, which manifest sweating, cold limbs, feeble and large or slow and weak pulse, add Radix Aconiti Praeparata to recuperate the depleted yang.
2. Applicable to cases of nocturnal emission with dizziness, fatigue, spiritlessness, reddish tongue, small and slow pulse, which are attributive to ineqilibri-

um between yin and yang.

3. Also applicable to cases of rheumatic heart disease, sinus bradycardia and atrioventricular block with palpitation, which are attributive to deficiency of heart-yang; and to cases of neurasthenia and hypogonadism with nocturnal emission, which are attributed to inequilibrium of yin and yang.

Interpretation

Glycyrrhizae is used in a large dose in this prescription and serves particulary to relieve palpitation and irritability. In sum, this prescription aims chiefly at warming and promoting heart-yang. Palpitation and other symptoms mentioned above may subside when the heart-yang is restored.

Decoction of Cinnamomi, Paeoniae and Aemarrhenae (Guizhi Shaoyao Zhimu Tang)

Ingredients

Ramulus Cinnamomi	10 g
Radix Paeoniae Alba	10 g
Rhizoma Zingiberis Recens	10 g
Rhizoma Atractylodis Macrocephalae	10 g
Radix Anemarrhenae	10 g
Radix Ledebouriellae	10 g
Radix Aconiti Praeparata	6 g
Herba Ephedrae	5 g
Radix Glycyrrhizae	3 g

Efficacy

Expelling wind and dampness, activating yang- energy, relieving arthralgia, regulating yin and clearing away heat, mainly for cases with severe and imgratory arthralgia with swelling and increased temperature of the affected joints, dizzines, fatigue, nausea, vomiting, emaciation, thin and yellow greasy fur on the tongue, rapid pulse, which are attributive to accumulation of wind and dampness with production of heat evil.

Indications

1. This prescription is suitable for arthralgia of wind-dampness type with formation of heat. It is not indicated for those cases with severe heat which manifest high fever, thirst, red tongue with yellow and dry fur, smooth and rapid bounding pulse.
2. Applicable to cases of apoplexy involving the meridians manifested by hemiplegia, rigidity of limbs, dizziness, thin and yellow greasy fur on the tongue, wiry pulse, which are attributive to prolonged retention of wind and phlegm-dampness in the meridians with transformation of heat.
3. Also applicable to cases of chronic gouty arthritis, rheumatic arthritis, periomarthritis, etc. attributive to accumulation of wind- dampness with trnasformation of heat; and to cases of sequela of cerebrovascular accident and rheumatic cerebrobvasculitis with hemiplegia, which are attributive to retention of wind and phlegm-dampness in the meridians.

Interpretation

Ramulus Cinnamomi, Ledebouriellae, Ephedrae and Atractylodis Macrocephalae are used together to eliminate wind-dampness from both superficies and interior. Paeoniae Alba and Anemarrhenae have the effects of regulating yin and clearing away heat. Aconiti serves to activate yang-energy, expel dampness and alleviate pain when it is used together with Ramulus Cinnamomi, Paeoniae Alba and Anemarrhenae. It is noteworthy that drugs of both hot and cold or yin and yang nature are used simultaneously in the prescription, and their actions are promoted each other instead of antagonized.

Antipyretic and Antitoxic Bolus
(Qingwen Jiedu Wan)

Ingredients

Folium Isatidis
Fructus Forsythiae
Radix Scrophulariae
Radix Trichosanthis
Radix Platycodi
Fructus Arctii
Radix Seu Rhizoma Notopterygii
Radix Angelicae Dahuricae
Radix Ledebouriellae
Radix Puerariae
Radix Scutellariae
Radix Bupleuri
Rhizoma Ligustici Chuanxiong
Radix Paeoniae Rubra
Radix Glycyrrhizae
Herba Lophatheri

Efficacy

Having antipyretic and antitoxic functions.
Honey boluses, 9 g each bolus; 10 boluses per box.

Indications

Influenza, marked by fever with chills, anhidrosis with headache, thirst and dry throat, aching pain of limbs. It is also used to treat swelling and pain of mumps.

Administration and Dosage

To be taken orally, one bolus each time, twice a day. For children, the doses should be correspondingly reduced.

Bolus of Calculus Bovis for Purging the Heart-Fire
(Niuhuang qingxin wan)

Ingredients

Calculus Bovis	0.75 g
Cinnabaris	4.5 g
Rhizoma Coptidis	15 g
Radix Scutellariae	9 g
Fructus Gardeniae	9 g
Radix Curcumae	6 g

Indications

Clearing away heat evil and toxic material, waking up patients from unconsciousness by eliminating phlegm; mainly for seasonal febrile diseases with heat evil involving the pericardium and the phlegm-heat evil stagnating in the heart, which are manifested by high fever, irritability, coma, delirium, red tongue with yellowish fur.

Bolus of Citri Grandis
(Juhe wan)

Ingredients

Semen Citri Grandis	30 g
Sargassum	10 g

Thallus Laminariae seu Eckloniae	10 g
Thallus Laminariae Japonicae	10 g
Fructus Meliae Toosendan	10 g
Cortex Magnoliae Officinalis	10 g
Semen Persicae	6 g
Caulis Akebiae	6 g
Radix Aucklandiae	6 g
Lignum Cinnamomi	3 g

Efficacy

Activating circulation of vital qi and blood, dredging the passage of yang-qi, promoting diuresis, dissolving phlegm and softening the hard lumps; mainly for swelling of scrotum due to phlegm-dampness, with pain referred to the abdomen, whitish and greasy fur on the tongue and wiry pulse.

Indications

1. This prescription is applicable to cases with persistent swelling of scrotum. For cases with severe pain, add **Radix Angelicae Sinensis** and **Radix Cyathulae** to eliminate blood stasis and relieving pain; for cases with cold pain, add **Fructus Foeniculi** and **Fructus Evodiae** to warm the liver and expel the cold evil. In cases of transformation to heat from cold-dampness with redness, swelling, itching or yellowish discharge over the scrotum and oliguria, subtract **Lignum Cinnamomi** and add **Cortex Phellodendri**, **Radix Gentianae**, to clear away heat and dampness.

2. For single or multiple, smooth, and painless goiters attributive to stagnation of vital qi and phlegm, subtract **Caulis Akebiae**, and **Meliae Toosendan** and add **Rhizoma Cyperi** and **Bulbus Fritillariae Thunbergii** to promote circulation of vital qi and eliminate phlegm.

3. For cases of breast nodules, unilateral or bilateral, round or oval, smooth or nodular, attributive to stagnation of vital qi and phlegm, subtract **Caulis Akebiae** and add **Fructus hordei Germinatus** (in a large dosage) and **Retinervus Citri Fructus** to disperse the depressed liver-qi and dissolving phlegm.

4. Also applicable to case of hydrocele of tunica vaginalis, varicocele of spermatic cord, thyroid adenoma, breast fibroadenoma, etc. attributive to stagnation of vital qi and phlegm.

Interpretation

Semen Citri Grandis, bitter in taste and warm in nature, is an agent for regulating vital qi, dispersing stagnation and relieving pain. *Meliae Toosendan*, *Aucklandiae*, *Aurantii Immaturus* and *Magnoliae Officinalis* have the effects of dispersing the depressed liver-qi, relieving pain and promoting diuresis. *Laminarriae seu Eckloniae*, *Sargassum* and *Laminariae japonicae* serve to soften hard lumps, dissolve phlegm and disperse stagnation. *Lignum Cinnamomi* together with *Persicae* and *Corydalis* can warm the meridians and activate blood circulation; while together with *Aucklandiae* can promote diuresis and lead the dampness downwards.

Bolus of Rhei and Eupolyphaga seu Steleophaga
(Dahuang zhechong wan)

Ingredients

Radix et Rhizoma Rhei (steamed)	8 g
Eupolyphaga seu Steleophaga	6 g
Radix Scutellariae	6 g
Radix Glycyrrhizae	6 g
Semen Persicae	6 g
Semen Armeniacae Amarum	6 g
Tabanus Bivittatus	6 g
Holotrichia Diomphalia	6 g
Radix Paeoniae Alba	12 g
Radix Rehmanniae	30 g
Dry Lacquer	3 g
Hirudo	8 set

Grind the above ingredients into powder and is prepared as boluses, taken with warm wine.

Efficacy

Eliminating blood stasis and masses, nourishing blood to promote tissue regeneration; mainly for consumptive diseases attributive to retention of blood stasis in the body, which are manifested by emaciation, abdominal fullness, anorexia, squamation and dryness of skin, blackish coloration around the eyes, petechiae on the tongue, wiry and unsmooth pulse, etc..

Indications

1. For cases with localized abdominal pain and tenderness, dry stools, dark purplish tongue, wiry and small, smooth pulse, which are attributive to stagnation of blood and vital energy, hyperactivity of evil and sthenia of healthy energy, the prescription may be used as an analgesic and blood-stasis eliminating agent.

2. Also indicated for cases of erysipelas of the leg with lymphangitis, dark reddish tongue, wiry and unsmooth pulse, which are attributive to obstruction of meridians by blood stasis and heat.

3. Applicable to cases of amenorrhea accompanied with localized aching and marked tenderness over the lower abdomen, emaciation, purplish spots at the margin of the tongue, wiry and small, unsmooth pulse, which are attibutive to the stagnation of liver-blood.

4. Also applicable to cases of cirrhosis of liver, pulmonary tuberculosis, gastric cancer, thrombophlebitis, osteomyelitis, etc., which are attributive to retention of blood stasis in the body or obstruction of the meridians by blood stasis and heat.

Interpretation

Rhei activates blood circulation and eliminates blood stasis; *Eupolyphaga seu Steleophaga* removes stagnated blood and eliminates masses. They act together to discharge the blood stasis with feces. *Tabanus Bivittatus*, *Holotrichia*

Diomphalia, *Lacquer*, *Persicae* and *Hirudo* are applied to activate blood circulation and dredge the passage of meridians, and also applied № 6 to open the stagnated lung-qi and promote blood circulation; they all serve to increase the effect of eliminating blood stasis. № 10, 9 and № 4 can nourish blood and vessels to support healthy energy. № 3 purges stagnancy-heat which may be formed by blood stasis. Wine serves to enhance the effect of other drugs.

Bolus of Six Drugs Including Rehmannia
(Liuwei dihuang wan)

Ingredients

Rhizoma Rehmanniae Praeparata	240 g
Fructus Corni	120 g
Rhizoma Dioscoreae	120 g
Rhizoma Alismatis	90 g
Poria	90 g
Cortex Moutan Radicis	90 g

Grind the drugs into fine powder and mix with honey to make boluses as big as the seed of *Chinese parasol*, to be administered orally 6-9 grams each time with warm boiled water or slight salt water, twice or three times a day. The drugs can also be decocted in water for oral administration with the dosage reduced in proportion as the original recipe.

Efficacy

Nourishing and enriching the liver and kidney.

Indications

Syndrome due to the deficiency of vital esence of liver and kidney with symptoms of weakness and soreness of waist and knees, vertigo, tinnitus, deafness, night sweat, emission as well as persistant opening of fontanel. Or the flaring up of sthenic fire resulting in symptoms such as hectic fever, feverish sensation in the palms and soles, diabetes or toothache due to fire of deficiency type, dry mouth and throat, red tongue with little fur, and thready and rapid pusle.

Since it tends to be greasy tonics, the recipe should be administered carefuly to patients with weakened function of the spleen in transporting and distributing nutrients and water.

In addition, the above recipe can be modified to treat many other disease indicating the syndrome due to the deficiency of vital essence of liver and kidney such as vegetative nerve functional disturbance, hypertension, arteriosclerosis, diabetes, chronic nephritis, hyperthyroidism, pulmonary tuberculosis, chronic urinary infection, bronchial asthma, amenorrhea, scanty menstruation, or infantile dysplasia and interlectual hypoevolutism.

Interpretation

Prepared *rhizome of rehmannia*, as the principal one, possesses the effect of nourishing the kidney-yin and supplementing the essence of life. As assistant drugs, *dogwood fruit*, sour in flavor and warm in nature, is used for nourishing the kidney and replenishing the liver, while dried *Chinese yam* for nourishing the kidney-yin and tonifying the spleen. The rest ingredients collectively play the role of adjuvant drus. *Oriental water plantain* coordinates with the principal drug in clearing the kidney and purging turbid evils, *moutan bark* cooperates with dogwood fruit in purging liver fire, and poria shares the effort together with dried *Chinese yam* to excrete dampness from the spleen. The whole recipe acts as both tonics and purgatives with tonifying effect dominant.

Clinically and experimentally, the recipe has the effects of nourishing the body and consolidating the constitution, inhibiting hypercatabolism, reducing excitement of the brain, adjusting endocrine function and vegetative nerve, lowering blood pressure and blood sugar, inducing diuresis, improving the function of the kidney as well as promoting the epithelial hyperplasia of the esophagus and preventing cancer, etc..

Bolus of Ten Powerful Tonics
(Shiquan dabu wan)

Ingredients

Radix Codonopsis Pilosulae
Rhizoma Atractylodis Macrocephalae
Poria
Radix Glycyrrhizae
Radix Angelicae Sinensis
Rhizoma Ligustici Chuanxiong
Radix Paeoniae Alba
Radix Rehmanniae Praeparata
Radix Astragali seu Hedysari
Cortex Cinnamomi

Honeyed boluses, 9 g each bolus, 10 boluses per box. To be taken orally, one bolus each time, twice or three times daily.

Efficacy

Warming and nourishing qi and blood.

Indications

Deficiency of both qi and blood marked by sallow complexion, short breath, palpitation, dizziness, spontaneous perspiration, mental fatigue, lassitude of the extremities, profuse menstruation. It also serves as a supporting drug to detoxicating drugs in the treatment of non-healing of ulcers due to deficiency of qi and blood.

Cow-bezoar Bolus for Clearing Away Heat of the Upper Part of the Body
(Niuhuang shang qing wan)

Ingredients

Calculus Bovis
Herba Menthae
Flos Schizonepetae
Radix Ligustici Chuanxiong
Fructus Gardeniae
Rhizoma Coptidis
Cortex Phellodendri
Radix Scutellariae
Radix et Rhizoma Rhei
Fructus Forsythiae
Radix Paeoniae Rubra
Radix Angelicae Sinensis
Radix Rehmanniae
Radix Platycodi
Gypsum Fibrosum
Borneolum
Radix Glycyrrhizae

Grind the above drugs into fine powder, mix it with honey and make them into boluses, 6 g each bolus, 10 boluses per box.

Administration and Dosage

To be taken orally, one bolus each time, twice a day.

Efficacy

Clearing away heat and purging pathogenic fire, dispelling wind and relieving pain.

Indications

The syndromes of excessive fire in the middle and upper parts of the human body or the attack of pathogenic wind and heat on the upper part of the body marked by headache, vertigo, conjunctival congestion, tinnitus, swelling and sore throat, ulcerations of the mouth and tongue, swelling and soreness of the gums, constipation and dry stool.

Cautions

Pregnant women should be careful when taking this medicine.

Decoction for Clearing Away Pestilent Factors and Detoxification
(Qingwen baidu yin)

Ingredients

Cornu Rhinocerotis	18-24 g; 9-15 g; 6-12 g
Rhizoma Coptidis	12-18 g; 6-12 g; 3-5 g
Fructus Gardeniae	6-9 g
Radix Platycodi	6-9 g
Radix Scutellariae	6-9 g
Rhizoma Anemarrhenae	6-9 g
Radix Paeoniae Rubra	6-9 g
Radix Scrophulariae	6-9 g
Fructus Forsythiae	6-9 g
Radix Glycyrrhizae	6-9 g
Cortex Moutan Radicis	6-9 g
Herba Lophatheri	6-9 g

Commonly Used Prescriptions

Efficacy

Clearing away heat evil and toxic materials, cooling blood and supporting yin; mainly fro cases of seasonal epidemic diseses attributive to hyperactivity of severe heat in qifen and xuefen, which are manifested by high fever, restlessness, or even mania and delirium, thirst, intense headache, purplish red eruptions, hematemesis, epistaxis, dry lips, crimson tongue, rapid pulse.

Indications

1. The prescription is widely applicable to cases of internal medicine and surgery.
2. For critical cases of furunculosis complicated by septicemia attributive to the attack of viscera by toxic material, add *Flos Lonicerae* and omit *Lophatheri* and *Scrophulariae*.
3. For cases with general aching, intense headache, lumbago, oliguria, high fever, irritability, which are attributive to the attack of fire and pestilent evil, omit *Platycodi* and *Glycyrrhizae* and add *Rhizoma Imperatae* to nourish yin and promote diuresis. Nowadays, it is also applied for cases of leptospirosis with the above symptoms.
4. For cases with discharge of fresh or darkish bloody stools, high fever, irritability, red tongue, dry lips, sunken and small, rapid pulse, which are attributive to severe attack of pestilent evil, omit *Glycyrrhizae*, *Platycodi*, *Lophatheri*, *Forsythiae* and add *Flos Carthami*. Nowadays, it is also applied for cases of necrotizing enterocolitis with the same mechanism.
5. Also applicable to epidmeic meningitis, scarlet fever, erysipelas of face, septicemia, etc. attributive to the attack of pestilent evil and hyperactivity of heat in qifen and xuefen.

Interpretation

This prescription is composed of the modificatins of *White tiger decoction*, *Decoction of Coptidis for Detoxification* and *Decoction of Cornu Rhioncerotis and Rehmanniae*. *Gypsum Fibrosum*, *Anemarrhenae*, *Glycyrrhizae* and

Lophatheri have the effect of clearing away sthenic heat in qifen. *Coptidis*, *Gardeniae*, *Scutellariae* and *Forsythiae* have the effects of puring fire and elimination toxic materials. *Cornu Rhinocerotis*, *Rehmanniae*, *Moutan Radicis*, *Paeoniae Rubra* and *Scrophulariae* have the effects of cooling blood and preserving ying. The combination of three prescriptions constituents a strong agent for clearing away heat evil and toxic material.

Decoction for Clearing Heat in Ying System
(Qing ying tang)

Ingredients

Cornu Rhinocerotis	2 g
Radix Rehmanniae	15 g
Radix Scrophulariae	9 g
Herba Lophatheri	3 g
Radix Ophiopogonis	9 g
Radix Salviae Miltiorrhizae	6 g
Rhizoma Coptidis	5 g
Flos Lonicerae	9 g
Fructus Forsythiae	6 g

All the above drugs are to be decocted in water for oral administration.

Efficacy

Clearing and dispelling pathogenic heat from ying system, nourishing yin and promoting blood circulation.

Indications

Invasion of ying system by pathogenic heat manifested by feverish body which is aggravated in the night, delirium, insomnia due to vexation, or by faint skin rashes, deep-red and dry tongue and rapid pulse.

The recipe can also be modified to deal with ying-syndrome occuring in epidemic encephalitis B, epidemic cerebrospinal meningitis, septicemia and other infectious diseases.

Interpretation

In the recipe, *Cornu Rhinocerotis*, being salty in flavour and cold in property, and *Radix Rehmanniae* being sweet in taste and cold in nature, both exert a role of a principal drug, having the effect of removing heat from ying and blood systems. *Scrophulariae* and *Ophiopogonis* together act as assistant drugs having the effect of nourishing yin and clearing heat. The rest share the role of adjuvant and guiding drugs. *Lophatheri*, *Ophiopogonis*, *Lonicerae* and *Forsythiae* are used to clear and dispel pathogenic heat from ying system through qi system, and *Salviae Miltiorrhizae* is used to promote blood circulation to remove blood stasis.

Clinically and Experimentally, it is ascertained that the recipe possesses the efficacies of relieving inflammation, bringing down fever, tranquilizing the mind, resisting bacteria and viruses, tonifying the heart, arresting bleeding improving immunologic function, promoting blood circulation and so on.

Cases with white and slippery coating of the tongue which suggests invasion by pathogenic dampness should not use recipe in case it encourages pathogenic dampness.

Decoction for Strngthening Middle Jiao and Benefiting Vital Energy
(Bu zhong yi qi tang)

Ingredients

Radix Astragali seu Hedysari	15 g
Radix Codonopsis Pilosulae	15 g
Radix Angelicae Sinensis	10 g
Rhizoma Atractylodis Macrodephalae	10 g
Exocarpium Citri Grandis	6 g
Radix Glycyrrhizae Praeparata	6 g

Rhizoma Cimicifugae	3 g
Radix Bupleuri	3 g
Fructus Ziziphi Jujubae	6 g
Rhizoma Zingiberis Recens	6 g

Decoct the above ingredients in a right amount of water for oral administration.

Efficacy

Strengthening spleen, benefiting qi, lifting up yang-qi, mainly for the cases with deficiency of spleen and stomach and collapse of middle-jiao energy, manifested by shortness of breath, disinclination for speaking, tiredness, weakness, or prolapse of rectum, or fever due to deficiency of qi, pale tongue with white fur, empty and weak pulse.

Indications

1. This prescription is originally applied to fever due to internal damage, and now commonly for prolapse of rectum, gastroptosis and prolapse of uterus due to deficiency and collapse of qi.

2. Applicable to cases of common cold with deficiency of qi manifesting lingering fever, profuse sweating, pale tongue and weak pulse.

3. Also applicable to cases of septicemia, pulmonary tuberculosis, aplastic anemia, leukemia and summer fever which are manifested by fever due to deficiency of qi.

Interpretation

Astragali seu Hedysari has the effects of tonifying and lifting up qi; № 2, 4 and № 6 have the effects of strengthening the spleen and regulating the stomach, helping № 1 to tonify qi. While № 7 and № 8 have the effects of leading the stomach-qi upward, helping № 1 to lift up qi. № 3 can nourish blood and help qi to flow toward its bases. The case with deficiency of qi usually suffers from stagnation of qi, so the prescription includes № 5, 10 and № 9 to regulate qi and the stomach.

Modern studies have confirmed that the recipe has the efficacies in improving the cellular immune function promoting metabolism, improving the excitement of cerebral cortex, promoting the tension of skeletal muscles, smooth muscles and supporting tissues; and promoting digestion and absorption.

Cautions

Patients with internal heat due to yin deficiency is prohibited from taking this recipe, and for those with the impairment of body fluid and qi after illness, it's better to prescribe this recipe together with other drugs.

Decoction of Arctii for Soothing Muscles
(Niubang jieji tang)

Ingredients

Fructus Arctii	12 g
Fructus Forsythiae	12 g
Radix Scrophulariae	12 g
Fructus Gardeniae	10 g
Cortex Moutan Radicis	10 g
Spica Prunellae	10 g
Herba Dendrobii	10 g
Herba Schizonepetae	6 g
Herba Menthae	3 g

Decoct the above ingredients in a right amount of water for oral administration.

Efficacy

Clearing away heat and toxic material, expelling wind from the body surface and reducing swelling; mainly for skin infection of the head and neck, accompanied with fever, chilliness, headache, dry mouth, oliguria with reddish urine, red tongue with yellow fur, smooth and rapid pulse, which are attributive to the attack of wind, fire, toxic material and heat.

Indications

1. Applicable to cases of common cold attributive to attack of exogenous wind-heat, which manifest as fever, chilliness, headache, sore-throat, thirst, thinyellow fur on the tongue, floating and rapid pulse.

2. For cases of measles with interrupted eruption, fever, chilliness, sneezing, cough, congestion of conjunctiva, lacrimation, thirst, red tongue with thin yellow fur, floating and rapid pulse, which are attributive to attack of heat and toxic material to the lung and stomach, and retention of the pathogens in the superficies.

3. Also to cases of hordeolum accompanied with fever, chilliness, headache, thirst, red tongue and rapid pulse, which are attributive to attack of heat and toxic material to the eyes.

4. For cases of upper respiratory viral infection and inffluenza attributive to the attack of exogenous wind-heat; and for cases of chalazion and tarsitis attributive to the attack of heat evil and toxic material attack to the eyes.

Interpretation

Arctii acts as the principal drug of the prescription, which can expel wind and heat, eliminate toxic material and relieve swelling. *Schizonepetae*, *Menthae* help *Arctii* to disperse wind-heat from the head and face. *Forsythiae*, *Prunellae*, *Moutan Radicis*, *Gardeniae* and *Scrophulariae*, when used together with *Schizonepetae* and *Menthae*, serve to eliminate heat and toxic material from the head and face, to expel wind from the body surface and to relieve swelling. Because the retention of heat and toxic material can damage the yin-fluid, *Dendrobii* is applied to nourish yin and promote the production of body fluid. When the body fluid is sufficient, the high body temperature may become normal.

Decoction of Coptidis for Detoxification
(Neishu huanglian tang)

Ingredients

Rhizoma Coptidis	9 g
Radix Scutellariae	9 g
Fructus Gardeniae	9 g
Fructus Forsythiae	9 g
Radix Angelicae Sinensis	9 g
Radix Paeoniae Alba	9 g
Radix Aucklandiae	6 g
Herba Menthae	3 g
Radix Platycodi	3 g
Radix Glycyrrhizae	3 g
Radix et Rhizoma Rhei	6 g

Decoct the above ingredients in a right amount of water for oral administration.

Efficacy

Clearing away heat and toxic material, activating blood circulation, relieving swelling and promoting bowel movement.

Indications

To cases of jaundice manifested by bright yellow coloration over the body, fever, thirst, oliguria, reddish urine, constipation, yellow and greasy fur on the tongue, wiry and rapid pulse, which are attributive to the accumulation of dampness-heat.

To cases of appendicitis, liver abscess and lung abscess, to cases of cellulitis, lymphadenitis and mastitis and to cases of acute cholecystitis, icterus infectious hepatitis and cholelithiasis with jaundice attributive to the attack of dampness-heat.

Interpretation

Coptidis, *Scutellariae* and *Gardeniae* have the effects of clearing away heat evil and toxic material from the interior. *Menthae*, *Forsythiae* and *Platycodi* enhance the effects of the above drugs. *Angelicae Sinensis*, *Paeoniae Alba* and *Aucklandiae* serve to promote the circulation of vital qi and blood, and relieve swelling and pain. *Arecae* and *Rhei* promote the circulation of vital qi and bowel movement to purge the fire from below. *Glycyrrhizae* serves to increase the effect of *Rhei*. In sum, this prescription is designed for eliminating heat and toxic material both from the interior and the superficies.

Decoction of Cinnamomi Adding Cinnamomi
(Guizhi jia gui tang)

Ingredients

Ramulus Cinnamomi	15 g
Radix Paeoniae Alba	10 g
Rhizoma Zingiberis Recens	10 g
Radix Glycyrrhizae Praeparata	6 g
Fructus Ziziphi Jujubae	8 pcs

Decoct the above ingredients in a right amount of water for oral administration.

Efficacy

Activating yang-energy, eliminating cold, lowering adverse rising qi; mainly for cases attributive to attack of exogenous cold and adverse rising of cold originally retained in the lower jiao, which manifest feeling of an air flow moving from the lower abdomen upward to the chest and throat, abdominal pain, vomiting, intolerance of cold, white and greasy fur on the tongue, wiry and tense pulse.

Indications

Applicable to cases attributive to accumulation of yin-cold in the collaterals of jueyin, which manifest induration, swelling and pain of the scrotum, preference for warmth and aversion to cold, cold feet, white and greasy fur on the tongue, sunken and wiry pulse.

For cases with palpitation, frightening, feeling of fullness over the chest, cold limbs, white and greasy fur on the tongue, which are attributive to hypofunction of heart-yang, increase the dosage of *Glycyrrhizae Praeparata*.

Also applicable to cases of spasmodic colon and gastro-intestinal neurosis attributive to adverse rising of interior cold accompanied with the attack of exogenous cold; to cases of indirect inguinal hernia and inguinal hernia attributive to the accumulation of yin-cold; and also to cases of sinus arrhythmia and atrioventricular block attributive to hypofunction of heart-yang.

Interpretation

This prescription is composed by adding an extra dose of *Ramulus Cinnamomi* or *Cortex Cinnamomi* to the *Decoction of Ramulus Cinnamomi*. *Ramulus Cinnamomi* is used to disperse cold from the superficies and to lower the adverse rising qi, and serves as the principal drug of the prescription for both symptomatic and causative treatment. *Paeoniae Alba* serves to regulate ying and wei and to promote diaphoresis when it is used together with *Ramulus Cinnamomi*. It can also relieve pain and prevent abnormal rising of liver-qi when it is used together with *Glycyrrhizae Praeparata*. *Zingiberis Recens* can clear away cold, promote sweating and lower the adverse rising qi when it combines with *Ramulus Cinnamomi*, and can regulate ying and wei and warm the spleen and stomach when it combines with *Ziziphi Jujubae*. *Glycyrrhizae Praeparata* used with *Ramulus Cinnamomi* can relieve abnormal throbbing.

Decoction for General Antiphlogistic
(Puji xiaodu yin)

Ingredients

Radix Scutellariae	15 g
Rhizoma Coptidis	15 g
Fructus Forsythiae	10 g
Radix Isatidis	10 g
Radix Scrophulariae	10 g
Fructus Arctii	10 g
Exocarpium Citri Grandis	6 g
Radix Glycyrrhizae	6 g
Radix Bupleuri	6 g
Radix Platycodi	6 g
Lasiosphaera seu Calvatia	3 g
Herba Menthae	3 g
Bombyx Batryticatus	3 g
Rhizoma Cimicifugae	3 g

Decoct the above ingredients in a right amount of water for oral administration.

Efficacy

Clearing away heat evil and toxic material, expelling wind evil from the body surface, relieving swelling; mainly for some epidemic diseases attributive to the accumulation of wind, heat and pestilent evil in the head and face, manifested by swelling, redness and pain over the face, chilliness, fever, sore-throat, reddish tongue with white and yellow fur, floating and rapid, strong pulse, etc..

Indications

1. This is a representative prescription for treating the epidemic diseases characterized by swelling and redness of face. When the superficies-syndrome has

subsided and heat-syndrome becomes prominent. *Menthae* and *Bupleuri* should be subtracted and *Flos Lonicerae* added.

2. Applicable to furunculosis of the face and head attributive to upward attack of heat evil and toxic material (usually add *Lonicerae* and *Herba Schizonepetae*, and subtract *Lasiosphaera seu Calvatia* and *Bupleuri*).

3. Also applicable to cases of acute tonsillitis, acute otitis media, acute lymphadentis, mumps, etc., attributive to accumulation of wind-heat and pestilent evil in the head. In cases of mumps complicated by orchitis, add *Fructus Meliae Toosendan* to purge the sthenic fire of liver meridian.

Interpretation

Scutellariae and *Coptidis* are used in large dose to clear away heat evil and toxic material from the upper jiao. *Forsythiae*, *Arctii*, *Bombyx Batryticatus* and *Menthae* serve to expel wind-heat evil from the upper jiao. *Scrophulariae* and *Isatidis* enhance the effects of *Scutellariae*, and *Coptidis*, *Lasiosphaera seu Calvatia*, *Platycodi* and *Glycyrrhizae* are assisted by *Arctii* and *Menthae* to ease the throat. *Exocarpium Citri Grandis* has the effects of regulating vital energy and helps above drugs to expel wind evil and relieve swelling. *Cimicifugae* and *Bupleuri* can expel wind-heat evil and helps the above drugs distributing to the head and face. This is a well-known prescription for clearing away heat evil and toxic material.

Decoction for Purging Liver-fire and Eliminating Dampness (Qing gan sheng shi tang)

Ingredients

Radix Scutellariae	10 g
Fructus Gardeniae	10 g
Radix Angelicae Sinensis	10 g
Radix Paeoniae Alba	10 g
Radix Trichosanthis	10 g

Radix Rehmanniae	20 g
Rhizoma Ligustici Chuanxiong	6 g
Radix Bupleuri	6 g
Radix Gentianae	6 g
Rhizoma Alismatis	6 g
Caulis Akebiae	6 g
Medulla Junci	3 g
Radix Glycyrrhizae	3 g

Decoct the above ingredients in a right amount of water for oral administration.

Efficacy

Clearing away heat and dampness, dispersing the stagnated liver-qi, alleviating pain, activating the circulation of blood and relieving swelling; mainly for cases of scrotitis with chilliness, fever, oliguria, red tongue with yellow and greasy fur, wiry and rapid pulse, which are attributive to downward attack of dampness-heat from the liver meridian and the stagnation of blood and toxic materials.

Indications

1. For cases with induration, pain and swelling of testis, erythema and hotness of the scrotum, accompanied with chilliness, fever, headache, thirst, oliguria with deep-colored urine, red tongue with yellow and greasy fur, wiry and rapid pulse, which are attributive to downward attack of dampness-heat to the collateral of "jueyin" and the stagnation of blood and toxic material, add *Fructus Meliae Toosendan*, or *Semen Citri Grandis*, and omit *Glycyrrhizae* and *Junci*.

2. Also applicable to cases of hydrocele of tunica vaginalis, varicocele of spermatic cord, orchitis, tuberculosis of testis, etc. attributive to downward attack of dampness-heat and stagnation of blood and toxic material.

Interpretation

This prescription is formed by adding *Ligustici Chuanxiong*, *Paeoniae Alba*, *Trichosanthis* and *Junci*, and omitting *Semen Plantaginis* from the *Decoction of Gentianae for purging liver-fire*. In this prescription, *Gardeniae*, *Scutellariae* and *Gentianae* serve to purge the heat-toxic material from the liver meridian, and *Akebiae*, *Junci* and *Alismatis* to eliminate the dampness-toxic material from the lower-jiao. *Angelicae Sinensis*, *Rehmanniae*, *Paeoniae Alba*, *Ligustici Chuanxiong* are used together with *Bupleuri* to activate blood circulation, relieve swelling, disperse the stagnated liver-qi and alleviate pain. *Trichosanthis* has the effects of clearing away heat and eliminating phlegm, and promotes the subsidence of swelling. *Glycyrrhizae* serves to clear away heat and toxic material.

Golden Lock Bolus for Keep Kidney Essence
(Jinsuo gu jing wan)

Ingredients

Semen Astragali Complanati	30 g
Semen Euryales	30 g
Semen Nelumbinis	30 g
Stamen Nelumbinis	15 g
Os Draconis	20 g
Concha Ostreae	20 g

Efficacy

Strengthening kidney essence and stopping nocturnal emission; mainly for cases with hypofunction of kidney, characterized by nocturnal emission, fatigue, sorenss of limbs, lumbago, tinnitus, pale tongue with whitish fur, small and weak pulse.

Indications

1. Applicable to deficiency of both kidney-yin and yang. For cases with deficiency of kidney-yin predominantly, add Fructus Ligustri Lucidi and Fructus Rosae Laevigatae, while for those with deficiency of kidney-yang predominantly, add Fructus Psoraleae and Pulvis of Cornu Cervi. It is not suitabld for nocturnal emission due to hyperactivity of "prime-minister" fire.

2. For cases of leukorrhagia with thin discharge, attributive to deficiency of spleen-yang and yin, omit Stamen Nelumbinis and add Poria and Rhizoma Atractylodis Macrocephalae (in large dosage) to invigorate the spleen and kidney).

3. Applicable to cases of neurasthenia with nocturnal emission, and cervicitis with leukorrhagia, which are attributive to hypofunction of kidney.

Interpretation

Complanati has the effects of invigorating kidney, supporting kidney essence and stopping nocturnal emission. *Semen Nelumbinis* and *Semen Euryales* serve to clear away heart-fire, benefit the kidney and keep heart-fire and kidney-water in balance. *Os Draconis*, *Concha Ostreae* and *Stamen Nelumbinis* can relieve nocturnal emission and calm the mental state. All the above drugs constituent a prescription effective for arresting nocturnal emission.

Zaizao Powder
(Zaizao san)

Ingredients

Radix Astragali seu Hedysari	12 g
Radix codonopsis Pilosulae	10 g
Ramulus Cinnamomi	6 g
Radix Paeoniae Alba	6 g
Radix Aconiti Praeparata	6 g
Rhizoma seu Radix Notopterygii	6 g

Radix Ledebouriellae	6 g
Rhizoma Ligustici Chuanxiong	6 g
Herba Asari	3 g
Radix Glycyrrhizae Praeparata	3 g
Rhizoma Zingiberis Recens	5 pcs
Fructus Ziziphi Jujubae	2 pcs

Efficacy

Supporting yang-qi to promote sweating, benefiting vital qi and expelling superficial evils from body surface; mainly for cases of common cold of wind-cold type with a yang-deficiency constitution, manifested by fever with predominant chilliness, headache, rigidity of neck, anhidrosis, cold limbs, tiredness, pale complexion, low voice, pale tongue with whitish fur, sunken and weak pulse or floating and large, weak pulse, etc..

Indications

1. Applicable to the early stage of pyogenic infection of skin, manifested by local swelling and pain but no erythema nor heat, with predominant fever, chilliness, anhidrosis, cold limbs, no thirst, thin and whitish fur on the tongue, floating and large, weak pulse, which are attributive to attack of exogenous wind-cold and deficiency of yang-qi in the body.

2. Also indicated for cases of arthralgia with wandering pain, chilliness, fever, anhidrosis, cold limbs, tiredness, flat taste of the mouth, floating and large, weak pulse, which are attributive to attack of wind-cold-dampness evil to a person with yang-deficiency constitution.

3. Also applicable to cases of upper respiratory infection, mumps, rheumatic fever, rheumatoid arthritis, carbuncle, furuncle, acute cellulitis, etc., marked by chilliness and fever, which are attributive to deficiency of yang-qi and the attack of exogenous wind-cold-dampness or wind-cold evil.

Interpretation

This prescription is characterized by simultaneous application of cold-expelling and yang-supporting drugs. *Ramulus cinnamomi*, *Notopterygii*, *Ledebouriellae*, *Asari*, *Ligustici Chuanxiong* and *Zingiberis Recens* are diaphoretics for expelling cold. If only diaphoretics are used for those cases with a yang-deficiency constitution, not only perspiration does not occur but also the deficiency of yang would be aggravated, or even yang exhaustion after profuse sweating may ensue. So *Astragali seu Hedysari* and *Codonopsis* are applied to benefit yang-qi, and *Aconiti* is helpful for strengthen yang and promoting sweating. *Paeoniae Alba* and *Ziziphi Jujubae* can nourish blood. When used together with *Astragali seu Hedysari*, *Paeoniae Alba* exerts an astringent effect to prevent over sweating.

Powder for Antiphlogosis
(Baidu san)

Ingredients

Rhizoma seu Radix Notopterygii	12 g
Radix Angelicae Pubescentis	12 g
Radix Bupleuri	10 g
Radix Peucedani	10 g
Rhizoma Ligustici Chuanxiong	10 g
Radix Codonopsis Pilosulae	6 g
Fructus Aurantii	6 g
Poria	6 g
Radix Platycodi	6 g
Radix Glycyrrhizae	3 g
Herba Menthae	3 g
Rhizoma Zingiberis Recens	3 pcs

Decoct the above ingredients in a right amount of water for oral administration.

Efficacy

Benefiting vital qi and expelling the evils from the body surface, eliminating the wind and dampness evil; mainly for cases with insufficiency of healthy qi and attacked by exogenous wind, cold and dampness evil, which are manifested by chilliness, fever, headache, no sweating, general aching, stuffy nose, heavy voice, productive cough, whitish and greasy fur on the tongue, floating and weak pulse, etc..

Indications

1. Applicable to skin infections which are attributive to wind-cold-dampness superficies-syndrome.

2. By adding *Fructus Forsythiae* and *Flos Lonicerae*, and omitting *Codonopsis Pilosulae*, another prescription named *Powder of Forsythiae for Antiphlogosis* is formed. It is indicated for the initial stage of skin infections attributive to virulent heat evil attacking the superficies.

3. By adding *Herba Schizonepetae* and *Radix Ledebouriellae* and omitting *Codonopsis Pilosulae*, *Zingiberis Recens* and *Menthae*, another prescription named *Powder of Schizonepetae and Ledebouriellae for Antiphlogosis* is formed. It is indicated for affections of exogenous wind, cold and dampness evil, which are manifested by chilliness, fever, heavy sensation of head and body, cough, heavy voice, white and greasy fur on the tongue, wiry and tense pulse, etc..

4. Also applicable to cases of influenza, emphysema complicated by infection, malaria, acute cellulitis, etc., which are attirbutive to the affection of wind, cold and dampness evil in cases of the insufficiency of healthy qi.

Interpretation

Notopterygii and *Angelicae Pubescentis* not only can disperse wind-cold evil, but also can eliminate dampness and relieve pain. The former distributes upwardly and the latter downwardly, and they act on the whole body when used together. A small amount of *Codonopsis Pilosulae* is applied together with *Bupleuri*, *Ligustici Chuanxiong*, *Zingiberis Recens* and *Menthae* to invigorate vital qi and expel the evil factors from the body surface by sweating. A small amount of *Poria* is applied together with those drugs of *Peucedani*, *Aurantii* and *Platycodi* to eliminate sputum and relieve cough. *Radix Glycyrrhizae* serves to regulate the other drugs. This prescription combines both tonics and diaphoretics together, and possesses the advantage of producing sweating but not damaging the healthy qi, and that of supporting the healthy qi but not retaining the evils.

Pill of Six Miraculous Drugs
(Liushen wan)

Ingredients

Margarita	4.5 g
Calculus Bovis	4.5 g
Moschus	4.5 g
Realgar	3 g
Borneolum Syntheticum	3 g
Venenum Bufonis	3 g

Coated with burnt herbal powder.

Efficacy

Clearing away heat and toxic material, relieving swelling and alleviating pain; mainly for cases of scarlet fever and tonsillitis with red tongue and rapid pulse, which are attributive to the accumulation of phlegm, fire and toxic material.

Indications

1. The prescription cannot be applied as a decoction for oral use. Some ingredients such as *Realgar* and *Venenum Bufonis* are poisonous, so it should not be taken in alrge dose nor for a long period and is contraindicated for pregnant women.

2. Applicable to carbuncle, furuncle, abscess of breast, and various local infection of unknown origin, which are attributive to accumulation of phlegm, fire and toxic material.

3. Also applicable to cases of pharyngitis, follicular stomatitis, mastitis, nasopharyngeal carcinoma, lung cancer, etc. which are attributive to accumulation of phlegm, fire and toxic material.

The recipe can be modified to deal with influenza, epidemic encephalitis \ - B, epidemic cerebrospinal meningitis, pneumonia and septicemia indicating excessive heat syndrome in the qi system, and also with the treatment of stomatitis, periodontitis, gastritis, diabetes and others which pertain to stomach heat syndrome.

Interpretation

Calculus Bovis, *Realgar* and *Venenum Bufonis* are principal drugs in the prescrription, which have strong and fast effect of eliminating toxic materials and dispersing the accumulation of evils. *Calculus Bovis* can eliminate heat-phlegm, *Realgar* can disperse the stagnated substance, and *Venenum Bufonis* can relieve swelling and alleviate pain. They all are potent agents for clearing away heat and dispelling toxic material, and serve as the principal drugs of the prescription. *Margarita* can clear away heart-fire and eliminate phlegm when it combines with *Calculus Bovis*. *Borneolum Syntheticum* can disperse heat and alleviate pain, and also increase the effect of the other drugs with it combining with *Moschus*. *Burnt herbal powder* has the effect of dispersing the stagnated substance and easing the throat, and is especially good for the infection of oral cavity. In sum, the prescription has a strong detoxifying and swelling-subsiding effect by utilizing the fragrant nature of the ingredients.

Cautions

It is not advisable for those whose exterior syndrome is not relieved, nor for those who have fever due to blood-deficiency or cold syndrome with pseudo-heat symptoms.

Decoction of Phragmitis
(Weijing tang)

Ingredients

Rhizoma Phragmitis	60 g
Semen Coicis	30 g
Semen Benincasae	30 g
Semen Persicae	10 g

Decoct the above ingredients in a right amount of water for oral administration.

Efficacy

Clearing away lung-heat and eliminating sputum, removing blood stasis and pus; mainly for cases of pulmonary abscess with expectoration of foul, purulent and bloody sputum, chest pain aggravated by coughing, red tongue with yellow, greasy fur, smooth and rapid pulse.

Indications

1. This is a typical prescription for pulmonary abscess. For cases without formation of pus, add *Radix Platycodi* and *Bulbus Fritillariae Cirrhosae* to enhance the effect of eliminating the sputum and the pus.
2. For cases of measles after the occurrence of skin eruptions, but still with fever, productive cough, red tongue with yellow greasy fur, smooth and rapid pulse, which are attributive to lung-heat, omit *Persicae* and add *Cortex Mori Radicis* and *Bulbus Fritillariae Thunbergii*.
3. Also applicable to cases of lobar pneumonia, bronchitis, whooping cough, etc. which are attributive to lung-heat.

Interpretation

Phragmitis has the effects of clearing away lung-heat and is the principal remedy for pulmonary abscess. *Benincasae* eliminates sputum and pus. *Coicis* clears away heat-evil and promotes diuresis. *Persciae* removes blood stasis and pus. All of these three seeds can also move the bowels and eliminate the pus and blood stasis through defecation. These constitute and ideal prescription for pulmonary abscess of sputum-heat pattern or sputum-blood-stasis pattern. The abscess can be dispersed when the pus is not yet formed, and the pus can be eliminated when the abscess is formed.

Powder of Lonicerae and Forsythiae
(Yinqiao san)

Ingredients

Flos Lonicerae	12 g
Fructus Forsythiae	12 g
Fructus Arctii	10 g
Semen Sojae Praeparatum	10 g
Rhizoma Phragmitis	10 g
Radix Platycodi	5 g
Herba Menthae	5 g
Herba Lophatheri	5 g
Radix Glycyrrhizae	5 g
Spica Schizonepetae	5 g

Efficacy

Expelling wind and heat evil, clearing away heat evil and toxic material; mainly for cases due to exogenous wind and heat evil, which are manifested by fever, mild chilliness, sore-throat, headache, thirst, red tip of the tongue with thin white fur or thin yellowish fur, floating and rapid pulse, etc..

Indications

1. The therapeutic principle of this prescription is reasonable, the concept of compatibility is strict and its curative effect is fruitful, and has become a typical recipe for common cold of wind-heat type. For cases with extreme thirst, add *Radix Trichosanthis* to promote the production of saliva and quench thirst; for cases with sore-throat, add *Radix Scrophulariae* to clear away the heat evil and ease the throat.

2. For the initial stage of measles attributive to stagnation of wind and heat evil in the superficies, which is manifested by fever, thirst and incomplete eruption, add *Radix Puerariae* to let out the eruptions.

3. For cases at the onset of skin infections attributive to super ficies-syndrome of wind-heat type, add *Herba Taraxaci* or *Folium Isatidis* to clear away heat evil and toxic material, and dispersing the accumulation of evils.

4. Also applicable to cases of acute tonsillitis, influenza, mumps, measles, encephalitis B epidemic meningitis and acute suppurative infection, which are attributive to wind-heat syndrome of the superficies.

Interpretation

Lonicerae and *Forsythiae* are selected as principal drugs which have mild action to let the evil out of the body and clear away heat evil and toxic material, so as to prevent the evil from attacking the interior. *Schizonepetae*, *Menthae* and *Sojae Praeparatum* can expel the evils from the surface of the body owing to their acrid flavour. *Arctii*, *Platycodi* and *Glycyrrhizae* have the effects of clearing away heat evil and toxic material to ease the throat. *Lophatheri* and *Phragmitis* have the effects of clearing away heat evil and promoting the production of body fluid to relieve thirst. This prescription constitutes an acrid-cool remedy by combining the drugs of clearing away heat evil and toxic material with those of expelling the evil from the body surface. This model of compatibility exerts a great influence upon the later generation, and many new set prescriptions for common cold are composed of its modifications.

Powder of Ledebouriellae for Dispersing the Superficies
(Fangfeng tongsheng san)

Ingredients

Radix Ledebouriellae	10 g
Fructus Forsythiae	10 g
Fructus Gardeniae	10 g
Herba Schizonepetae	6 g
Herba Ephedrae	6 g
Rhizoma Ligustici Chuanxiong	6 g
Radix Angelicae Sinensis	6 g
Radix Paeoniae Alba	6 g
Rhizoma Atractylodis Macrocephalae	6 g
Radix et Rhizoma Rhei	6 g
Natrii Sulfas	6 g
Radix Scutellariae	6 g
Talcum	20 g
Gypsum Fibrosum	15 g
Herba Menthae	3 g
Radix Platycodi	3 g
Radix Glycyrrhizae	3 g
Rhizoma Zingiberis Recens	3 pcs

Decoct the above ingredients in a right amount of water for oral administration.

Efficacy

Expelling wind from the body surface, clearing away heat and promoting bowel movement; mainly for sthenia-syndrome of both the superficies and the interior after the attack of exogenous wind-heat and the retention of heat in the interior, which is manifested by aversion to cold, fever, dizziness, bitter and dry mouth, conjunctivitis, sore-throat, feeling of oppression over the chest, constipation, dysuria with reddish urine, red tongue with white or yellow fur, floating and smooth, rapid pulse.

Indications

1. Applicable to cases of early stage of superficial pyogenic infection with local signs of inflammation, chilliness, fever, bitter mouth, constipation, oliguria, red tongue with white fur, floating and rapid pulse.

2. Also indicated for cases of urticaria and eczema with thin and white fur on the tongue, floating and rapid pulse, which are attributive to simultaneous existence of sthenia-syndrome in the superficies and the interior.

3. Also applicable to cases of influenza, poliomyelitis, infectious mononucleosis, mumps, acute cellulitis, erysipelas, acute lymphangitis, etc., which are attributive to simultaneous existence of sthenia-syndrome in the superficies and the interior after attack of exogenous wind-heat and retention of heat in the body.

Interpretation

Ledebouriellae, *Schizonepetae*, *Ephedrae*, *Zingiberis Recens* and *Menthae* serve to expel wind by sweating. *Rhei* and *Natrii Sulfas* eliminate the internal heat by purgation, and *Gardeniae* and *Talcum* clear away heat by diuresis. *Platycodi*, *Gypsum Fibrosum*, *Scutellariae* and *Forsythiae* can clear away heat from the lung and stomach. All the above drugs act together to eliminate heat from the upper and the lower part of the body, and treat both the superficies and the interior syndrome. *Angelicae Sinensis*, *Ligustici Chuanxiong* and *Paeoniae Alba* have the effects of expelling wind and nourishing blood, and *Atractylodis Macrocephalae* and *Glycyrrhizae* serve to strengthen the spleen and regulating the stomach; they cooperate each other to exert a diaphoretic effect without damaging the superficies, and exert a purgative effect without impairing the interior. In sum, this prescription involves the therapeutic principles of diaphoretic, heat-eliminating, purgative and tonifying simultaneously, aiming at clearing away the internal heat chiefly. The application of *Natrii Sulfas* and *Rhei* is for purging heat.

White Tiger Decoction
(Baihu tang)

Ingredients

Gypsum Fibrosum	30 g
Rhizoma Anemarrhenae	9 g
Radix Glycyrrhizae Praeparata	3 g
Semen Oryzae Nonglutionosae	9 g

All the above drugs are to be decocted in water for oral administration.

Efficacy

Clearing away heat and promoting the production of body fluid.

Indications

Yangming channel diseases marked by high fever, flushed face, polydipsia, profuse perspiration, aversion to heat and full forceful pulse. It can be modified to treat influenza, epidemic encephalitis B, epidemic cerebrospinal meningitis, pneumonia and septicemia indicating excessive heat syndrome in the qi system.

Cautions

It is not advisable for those whose exterior syndrome is not relieved, nor for those who have fever due to blood-deficiency or cold syndrome with pseudo-heat symptoms.

Decoction of Gypsum Fibrosum and Three Yellows
(Sanhuang shigao tang)

Ingredients

Gypsum Fibrosum (decocted first	30 g
Radix Scutellariae	10 g
Rhizoma Coptidis	10 g
Cortex Phellodendri	10 g
Fructus Gardeniae	10 g
Semen Sojae Praeparatum	10 g
Herba Ephedrae	3 g
Rhizoma Zingiberis Recens	3 pcs
Fructus Ziziphi Jujubae	2 pcs
Folium Camelliae Sinensis	6 g

Decoct the above ingredients in a right amount of water for oral administration.

Efficacy

Expelling the pathogens from both the interior and the superficies, purging fire and eliminating toxic materials; mainly for seasonal febrile diseases involving both the interior and superficies, which manifest as high fever, chilliness, anhidrosis, flushed cheeks, dryness of teeth and nose, extreme thirst, severe headache, irritability or even mania, red tongue with yellow fur, bounding and rapid or smooth and rapid pulse.

Indications

1. For cases with yang macules which are punctate or pieces and bright red in colour, accompanied with high fever, thirst, flushed cheeks, conjunctival congestion, red or crimson tongue with yellow fur, bounding and rapid pulse, which are attributive to stagnation of heat in the *yangming* channel involving *yingfen* and *xuefen*, use *Radix Rehmanniae* instead of *Ephedrae* and *Sojae Praepara-*

tum.

2. Also applicable to cases suffering from common cold, encephalitis B, typhoid fever and paratyphoid fever with high fever, which are attributive to attack of potent heat to both interior and the superficies; and to cases of epidemic hemorrhagic fever, typhus fever, which are attributive to the stagnation of heat in the *yangming* channel involving *yingfen* and *xuefen*.

3. Applicable to infections of skin and subcutaneous tissues acccompanied with high fever, irritability, extreme thirst, oliguria with reddish urine, red tongue with yellow fur, wiry and rapid pulse, which are attributive to retnetion of heat and toxic material in the superficies when the pathogens are potent and the healthy energy is still strong.

Interpretation

Gypsum Fibrosum can clear away the interior heat and acts as the chief drug of the prescription. *Ephedrae* and *Sojae Praeparatum* are applied to promote sweating and discharge the heat outside. The above three durgs used together can expel heat from both the interior and the superficies. Since there is a large amount of heat in the triple-jiao, *Scutellariae* is applied to clear away the heat in the upper-jiao. *Gardeniae* and *Camelliae Sinensis* can discharge the heat of triple-jiao from the urine. *Zingiberis* and *Ziziphi Jujubae* serve to regulate *ying* and *wei*.

Decoction of Ginseng for Nourishing Qi and Ying
(Renshen yang rong tang)

Ingredients

Radix Paeoniae Alba	15 g
Radix Rehmanniae Praeparata	15 g
Radix Codonopsis Pilosulae	10 g
Radix Astragali seu Hedysari	10 g
Rhizoma Atractylodis Macrocephalae	10 g

Poria	10 g
Radix Angelicae Sinensis	10 g
Exocarpium Citri Grandis	6 g
Fructus Schisandrae	6 g
Radix Glycyrrhizae Praeparata	3 g
Cortex Cinnamomi	3 g
Radix Polygalae	3 g
Rhizoma Zingiberis Recens	3 pcs
Fructus Ziziphi Jujubae	3 pcs

Decoct the above ingredients in a right amount of water for oral administration.

Efficacy

Benefiting qi, tonifying blood, strengthening spleen and nourishing heart; mainly for consumptive diseases manifested by palpitation, amnesia, insomnia, dreaminess, tiredness, profuse sweating, poor appetite, shortness of breath, dyspnea upon exertion, pale tongue, sunken and weak pulse, which are attributive to insufficiency of qi and blood, and hypofunction of heart and spleen.

Indications

Applicable to cases of irregular (or delayed) menstruation with scanty pale discharge, sallow complexion, palpitation, dizziness, shortness of breath, fatigue, poor appetite, pale tongue, which are attributive to deficiency of liver-blood and spleen-qi and failure of releasing stagnated qi and controlling blood.

2. Also indicated for the late stage of pyogenic infection of skin when the acute inlammation subsides but the qi and blood are deficient, which manifest lesion with discharge of thin purulent fluid, dark greyish coloration but without granulation, and accompanied with lusterless complexion and pale tongue.

3. Also applicable to cases of pulmonary tuberculosis, rheumatic heart diseases, gastric ulcer, tuberculous abscess, carbuncle, phlebeurysma of the lower limbs, etc. which are attributive to deficiency of qi and blood.

Interpretation

The prescription is composed by omitting *Rhizoma Ligustici Chuanxiong* and adding *Astragali seu Hedysari*, *Cortex Cinnamomi*, *Citri Grandis*, *Schisandrae* and *Polygalae* to the *Decoction of Eight Ingredients for Tonifying Qi and Blood*. *Ligustici Chuanxiong* is omitted because the effect of activating blood circulation is not desired. The effect of tonifying blood and promoting blood production is obtained when *Astragali seu Hedysari* is used together with *Angelicae Sinensis*. *Cortex Cinnamomi* used together with *Zingiberis Recens*, *Ziziphi Jujubae* can accelerate the growth of qi and blood. *Polygalae* and *Schisandrae* adding to *Codonopsis Pilosulae* and *Astragali seu Hedysari* serve to benefit the heart-qi and tranquilizing. *Citri Grandis* is used for regulating qi and stomach to decrease the indigestibility of the tonics.

Ease Powder
(Xiao Yao San)

Ingredients

Radix bupleuri	15 g
Radix Angelicae Sinensis	15 g
Radix Paeoniae Alba	15 g
Poria	15 g
Rhizoma Atractylodis Macrocephalae	15 g
Rhizoma Zingiberis Recens Praeparata	3 g
Herba Menthae	3 g
Radix Glycyrrhizae Praeparata	6 g

Grind the above drugs except *ginger* and *peppermint* into powder take 6 to 9 grams each time with a decoction in small amount of roasted *ginger* and *peppermint*.

Efficacy

Soothing the liver disperse depressed qi, and invigorating the spleen to nourish the blood.

Indications

Stagnation of the liver-qi with deficiency of the blood marked by hypochondriac pain, headache, dizziness, bitter mouth, dry throat, mental weariness and poor appetite, or alternate attacks of chills and fever, or irregular menstruation, distension in the breast, light redness of the tongue, taut and feeble pulse.

Patients with chronic hepatitis, Pleuritis, chronic gastritis, neurosis, irregular menstruation marked by symptoms of stagnation of liver-qi with deficiency of the blood can be treated by the modified recipe.

Interpretation

Bupleurum root in the recipe soothes the liver to disperse the depressed qi. *Chinese yam* and *White peony root* nourish the blood and the liver. The joint use of the three drugs is able to treat the primary cause of stagnation of the liver-qi and deficiency of the blood. *Poria* and *Bighead atractylodes rhizome* strengthen the middle-jiao and reinforce the spleen so as to enrich the source of growth and development of the qi and blood. *Roasted ginger* regulates the stomach and warms the middle-jiao. *Peppermint* assists *Bupleurum root* in soothing the liver to disperse the depressed qi. *Prepared licorice root* can not only assist *Bighead atractylodes rhizome* and *Poria* in replenishing qi and invigorating the middle-warmer but also coordinate the effects of all the drugs in the recipe.

Modern researches have proved that the recipe has remarkable effects of nourishing the liver, tranquilizing the mind and relieving spasm. It is also effective in promoting digestion, coordinating uterine function, nourishing blood, strengthening the stomach and so on.

Decoction of Aneglicae Pubescentis and Taxilli
(Duhuo Jisheng Tang)

Ingredients

Radix Angelicae Pubescentis	10 g
Cortex Eucommiae	10 g
Radix Achyranthis Bidentatae	10 g
Radix Gentianae Macrophyllae	10 g
Poria	10 g
Radix Ledebouriellae	10 g
Radix Angelicae Sinensis	10 g
Radix Codonopsis Pilosulae	10 g
Radix Paeoniae Alba	10 g
Ramulus Taxilli	18 g
Radix Rehmanniae	18 g
Lignum Cinnamomi	1.5 g
Rhizoma Ligustici Chuanxiong	6 g
Herba Asari	3 g
Radix Glycyrrhizae	3 g

Decoct the above ingredients in a right amount of water for oral administration.

Efficacy

Expelling wind-dampness evil, relieving arthralgia, benefiting the liver and kidney, invigorating vital energy and blood; mainly for prolonged arthralgia of wind-cold- dampness type with hypofunction of liver and kidney and insufficiency of vital energy and blood, which is manifested as cold pain over the loin and joints, limited mobility and flaccidity of joints, or numbness, aversion to cold and desire for warmth, pale tongue with whitish fur, small and weak pulse.

Indications

1. Applicable to cases of stroke manifested by hemiplegia, numbness, spasm of limbs, pale tongue with whitish fur, small and weak pulse, which are attributive to deficiency of both the liver and the kidney, and attack of wind evil to the meridians.

2. Also applicable to cases of chronic rheumatic arthritis, rheumatic sciatica, lumbar strain, prolapse of lumbar intervertebral disc, etc., marked by cold pain over the loin and knees, which are attributive to prolonged bi-syndrome with deficiency of both the liver and the kidney and insufficiency of vital energy and blood.

Interpretation

Angelicae Pubescentis, *Ledebouriellae* and *Gentianae Macrophyllae* have the effects of expelling wind and dampness, *Asari* expels wind-cold evil from the yin-channel and eliminates wind-dampness evil from the muscles and tendons; the above three drugs used together exert an analgesic effect for rheumatism of wind-cold-dampness type evil and relieving pain. Prolonged rheumatism (attack of wind-cold-dampness evil) may aggravate the deficiency of liver and kidney, so *Ramulus Taxilli*, *Achyranthis Bidentatae* and *Eucommiae* are applied to tonify the liver and kidney, strengthen the tendons and bones, *Codonopsis Pilosulae*, *Poria*, *Glycyrrhizae* to invigorate healthy energy, and *Rehmanniae*, *Angelicae Sinensis* and *Paeoniae Alba* to nourish blood and activate blood circulation. Moreover, *Ligustici Chuanxiong* and *Lignum Cinnamomi* are added to warm and dredge the vessels and expel wind evil. In sum, the prescription serves as both symptomatic and causative therapy for arthralgia by supplementing vital energy and blood, invigorating liver and kidney, and eliminating wind.

Decoction for Pus Drainage and Relieving Pain
(Tuoli ding tong tang)

Ingredients

Radix Rehmanniae Praeparata	18 g
Radix Angelicae Sinensis	12 g
Radix Paeoniae Alba	12 g
Rhizoma Ligustici Chuanxiong	8 g
Pericarpium Papaveris	8 g
Cortex Cinnamomi	3 g
Olibanum	3 g
Myrrhae	3 g

Decoct the above ingredients in a right amount of water for oral administration.

Efficacy

Nourishing blood, promoting granulation, eliminating blood stasis and relieving pain; mainly for unhealed carbuncle after rupture with thin purulent bloody discharge, severe pain, poor granulation, pale tongue, small and rapid pulse.

Indications

1. Applicable to cases of dysmenorrhea with oligomenorrhea and darkish discharge, fatigue, pale or darkish tongue, sunken and small, unsmooth pulse, which are attributive to deficiency and stagnation of blood.

2. Also applicable to cases of thromboangiitis obliterans, chronic ulcer of lower extremity and tuberculosis of cervical lymph nodes with unhealed wound and poor granulation and case of endometriosis, endometritis, hysteromyoma and vegetative neurosis marked by dysmenorrhe, which are attributive to deficiency and stagnation of blood.

Interpretation

Olibanum and *Myrrhae* promote blood circulation and remove blood stasis to relieve pain. *Rehmanniae Praeparata*, *Angelicae Sinensis*, *paeoniae Alba* and *Ligustici Chuanxiong* are used for nourishing blood to promote granulation and help the first two drugs to promote blood circulation and relieve pain. A small dosage of *Cinnamomi* combined with *Rehmannaie Praeparata* and *Angelicae Sinensis* has the effects of activating the blood and vital qi circulation and promoting granulation. *Pericarpium Papaveris* exerts a prompt astringent and analgesic effect.

Xiaojin Pellet
(Xiao jin dan)

Ingredients

Resina Liquidambaris	3 g
Radix Aconiti Kusnezoffii	6 g
Olibanum	6 g
Myrrha	6 g
Faeces Trogropterori	10 g
Radix Angelicae Sinensis	10 g
Lumbricus	10 g
Carbonized Chinese ink	1 g

The above drugs are ground into powder and prepared as pellets, taken with rice wine.

Efficacy

Eliminating cold, expelling phlegm, removing blood stasis and reducing swelling; mainly for multiple abscesses, subcutaneous nodules, scrofula, and osteomyelitis with local pain and swelling, which are attributive to retention of phlegm-dampness evil in the meridians.

Indications

1. Applcable to cases of stomachache with tenderness, or hematemesis with purplish-dark discharge, darkish tongue with white and smooth fur, unsmooth pulse, which are attributive to stagnation of blood and phlegm.
2. Also applicable to cases of cold abscess, tuberculous lymphadenitis, tuberculosis of joints and chronic osteomyelitis attributive to the stagnation of cold-phlegm and dampness; also to cases of gastric cancer and breast carcinoma attribvutive to the stagnation of blood and phlegm.

Interpretation

Aconit Kusnezoffii has the effects of eliminating cold and dampness, dredging the passage of meridians, reducing swelling and alleviating pain. *Momordicae and Resina Liquidambaris* serve to reduce swelling and alleviate pain. *Moschus* can reopen the meridians, remove blood stasis and relieve swelling. The above four drugs serve as the principal drugs in the prescription. *Lumbricus* used together with *Aconiti Kusnezoffii* can eliminate phlegm and cold, dredge the passage of meridians and activate yang. *Carbonized Chinese ink* used together with *Moschus* can eliminate dampness, remove blood stasis and reduce swelling. *Olibanum*, *Myrrha*, *Faeces Trogopterori* and *rice wine* can activate blood circulation, reduce swelling and alleviate pain. *Angelicae Sinensis* is applied for nourishing blod, so that the healthy qi will not be impaired when blood stasis is removed by other drugs. It also enhances the effect of *Aconiti Kusnezoffii*.

Decoction for Warming Yang
(Yang he tang)

Ingredients

Radix Rehmanniae Praeparata	30 g
Cortex Cinnamomi	3 g
Herba Ephedrae	2 g

Colla Cornus Cervi	9 g
Semen Sinapis Albae	6 g
Rhizoma Zingiberis Praeparata	2 g
Radix Glycyrrhizae	3 g

Decoct the above ingredients in a right amount of water for oral administration.

Efficacy

Warming yang, tonifying blood, expelling cold and dispersing stagnation; mainly for yin type carbuncle, bone carbuncle, multiple abscesses and arthroncus of knee joint, attributive to deficiency of blood and stagnation of cold evil, manifested by local and not well-demarcated swelling, no change of color and temperature, no pain or just mild aching, pale tongue with whitish and smooth fur, sunken and slow pulse.

Indications

1. For cases of yin type carbuncle with pale tongue, floating and large pulse, complicated by deficiency of vital qi, add raw **Radix Astragali seu Hedysari** to benefit vital qi and promot pus drainage.

2. Applicable to cases of dyspneic cough with profuse and thin sputum, which are attributive to hypofunction of both lung and kidney with retention of dampness-phlegm, in this case the prescription is used for warming and invigorating the lung and kidney, eliminating sputum and relieving dyspnea. It may also be applied for cases of bi-syndrome and dysmenorrhea attributive to blood deficiency and cold-stagnation, and serves to warm yang, tonify blood, expel cold evil and arrest pain in this case.

3. Also applicable to cases of deep abscess, bone tuberculosis, chronic osteomyelitis, rheumatic arthritis, tuberculosis of knee joint, etc. which are attributive to blood-deficiency and cold-stagnation.

Interpretation

Rehmanniae Praeparata has the effcts of warming and tonifying ying-blood and inhibiting diaphoretic effect of *Ephedrae*, so that the latter preserves the action of warming the striae. *Colla Cornus Cervi* can produce essence substance, nourish bone marrow and blood, and support yang. It also inhibits the "dispersing" effect of *Cinnamomi* and *Zingiberis* and renders them just for warming and dredging the channels, and removing the stagnation of cold and phlegm. In turn, *Cinnamomi* and *Zingiberis* render *Rehmanniae Praeparata* and *Colla Cornus Cervi* exerting tonic effect but not greasy. *Ephedrae* distributes to the superficis, while *Rehmanniae Praeparata* to the interior. Two drugs help each other to warm and dredgethe striae and channels. *Sinapis Albae* serve to eliminate phlegm and disperse the stagnation of evil. *Glycyrrhizae* is used rawly just for detoxification. In summary, this prescription does not stress on the elimination of toxic material for the treatment of yin type carbuncle. It composed of drugs for warming yang, nourishing blood, dispersing cold and dredging stagnation of evil, thus embodies the therapeutic principle that the root cause of the disease must be aimed at.

Decoction of Persicae for Purgation
(Taohe chengqi tang)

Ingredients

Semen Persicae	12 g
Radix et Rhizoma Rhei	12 g
Ramulus Cinnamomi	10 g
Radix Glycyrrhizae Praeparata	6 g
Natrii Sulfas	6 g

Decoct the above ingredients in a right amount of water for oral administration.

Efficacy

Eliminating blood stasis and purging heat evil; mainly for blood-stagnation syndrome due to accumulation of blood stasis and heat evil in the lower jiao, which is manifested by distending pain over the lower abdomen, irritability, sunken and solid pulse.

Indications

1. For cases of preceded menstrual cycle, amenorrhea, metrorrhagia, etc., attributive to combination of blood stasis and heat evil in the lower jiao, omit *Glycyrrhizae* from the prescription and add *Radix Angelicae Sinensis* to regulate meenstruation, activate blood circulation, eliminate blood stasis and stop bleeding.

2. For cases of abdominal pain after operation due to blood stasis, or trauma (especially the early stage of fracture of thoracic or lumbar vertebrae), which are attributive to combination of blood stasis and heat evil, omit *Glycyrrhizae* and add *Radix Cyathulae* to activate blood circulation and eliminate blood stasis, and let the blood flowing downwards.

3. Applicable to cases of hematemesis, headache, congestion of conjunctiva, which are attributive to upward attack of blood stasis and heat evil.

4. Also applicable to cases of intestinal obstruction, pelvic cellulitis, appendicitis, etc. with abdominal pain, or cases of retention of placenta, dysfunctional uterine bleeding, etc. with headache or bleeding from the gum, which are attributive to combination or upward attack of blood stasis and heat evil.

Major Decoction for Purging Down Digestive Qi
(Da chengqi tang)

Ingredients

Radix et Rhizoma Rhei	12 g
Cortex Magnoliae Officinalis	15 g

Fructus Aurantii Immaturus	12 g
Natrii Sulfas	9 g

Decoct the above ingredients in a right amount of water for oral administration.

Efficacy

Expelling pathogenic heat and loosening the bowel, promoting the circulation of qi to purge accumulation in the bowels.

Indications

1. Excessive-heat syndrome of *yangming-fu* organ, manifested by constipation, frequent wind through the anus, feeling of fullness in the abdomen, abdominal pain with tenderness and guarding, tidal fever, delirium, polyhidrosis of hands and feet, prickled tongue with yellow dry fur or dry black tongue coating with fissures, deep and forceful pulse.

2. Syndrome of fecal impaction due to heat with watery discharge, manifested by watery discharge of terribly foul odor accompnaied by abdominal distension and pain with tenderness and guarding, dry mouth and tongue, smooth and forceful pulse.

3. Cold limbs due to excess of heat, convulsion, mania and other symptoms belonging to excess syndrome of interior heat.

Equally, this recipe can be modified to deal with infectious or non-infectious febrile diseasesin their climax marked by accumulation of heat type, and in the treatment of paralytic, simple and obliterative intestinal obstructions.

Interpretation

Rhei has the purgative effect and eliminating heat, but cannot induce an immediate purgation since it only promotes the peristalsis of large intestine and cannot soften the dry feces. While *Natrii Sulfas* can creat a hypertonic condition in the large intestine and retain enough amount of water to softne the dry feces. hence the two drugs used together may give an immediate purgation. Moreover,

Magnoliae Officinalis and *Aurantii Immaturus* have the effects of promoting vital qi circulation and relieving distension in the abdomen, so as to regulate the function of the gastrointestine, and enhance the effect of *Rhei* and *Natrii Sulfas*.

Major Decoction of Bupleurum
(Da chaihu tang)

Ingredients

Radix Bupleuri	15 g
Radix Scutellariae	9 g
Radix Paeoniae Alba	9 g
Rhizoma Pinelliae	9 g
Fructus Aurantii Immaturus Praeparata	9 g
Radix et Rhizoma Rhei	6 g
Rhizoma Zingiberis Recens	15 g
Fructus Ziziphi Jujubae	5 pcs

Decoct the above ingredients in a right amount of water for oral administration.

Efficacy

Treating *shaoyang* disease by mediation and purging away internal stasis of heat.

Indications

Shaoyang and *yangming* diseases complex marked by alternate attacks of chills and fever, fullness and oppression in the chest, hypochondriac discomfort, frequent vomiting, mental depression and dysphoria, epigastric fullness and pain or epigastric rigidity, constipation or diarrhea due to interior cold and exterior heat, yellow tongue fur, stringy and forceful pulse.

Patients with acute cholecystitis, cholelithiasis, acute pancreatitis and infection of abdominal activity marked by the above-mentioned symptoms can be treated by the modified recipe.

Pill of Stephaniae Tetrandrae, Zanthoxyli, Lepidii seu Descurainiae and Rhei
(Ji jiao li huang wan)

Ingredients

Radix Stephaniae Tetrandrae	10 g
Semen Zanthoxyli	10 g
Semen Lepidii seu Descurainiae	10 g
Radix et Rhizoma Rhei	6 g

Decoct the above ingredients in a right amount of water for oral administration.

Efficacy

Eliminating the retained fluid and discharging the evils from the lower part; mainly for phlegm-retention syndrome manifested by abdominal fullness, loose stools, dry mouth and tongue, sunken and wiry pulse, which is attributive to retention of fluid in the intestines when the healthy energy is still strong and the evil is hyperactive.

Indications

1. Applicable to cases of dyspneic cough accompanied by feeling of fullness over the chest, inability to lie flat, profuse expectoration, constipation, oliguria, yellow and greasy fur, wiry and smooth pulse, which are attributive to retention of fluid in the thorax.

2. Also inidcated for cases of dysuria accompanied with dyspnea, constipation, floating and smooth pulse, which are attributive to stagnation of phlegm-

heat in the lung, and adverse rising of qi.

3. Also applicable to cases of cirrhosis of liver, chronic nephritis, idiopathic edema, tuberculous pleurisy, lung cancer with pleuralmetastasis, acute glomerular nephritis, urinary infection, etc. which are attributive to fluid or phlegm retention.

Powder of Bupleuri for Dispersing the Depressed Liver-Qi
(Chaihu shugan san)

Ingredients

Radix Bupleuri	10 g
Fructus Aurantii	10 g
Rhizoma Ligustici Chuanxiong	10 g
Exocarpium Citri Grandis	10 g
Rhizoma Cyperi	10 g
Radix Paeoniae Alba	15 g
Radix Glycyrrhizae Praeparata	6 g

Decoct the above ingredients in a right amount of water for oral administration.

Efficacy

Dispersing the stagnated liver-qi, regulating vital qi, activating blood circulation and relieving pain; mainly for ceses due to stagantion of liver-qi and vital qi manifested by fullness of breast, hypochondriac pain, or dysmenorrhea, or stomachache, and for cases due to stagnation of liver and gallbladder heat manifested by alternating episodes of chills and fever.

Indications

1. This prescription and *Powder for Treating Yang Exhaustion* both have the similar action and indication, but the former, owning to the action of *Bupleuri*,

ahs a stronger effect on dispersing the stagnated liver-qi, regulating the vital qi and adtivating blood circulation. It is frequently applied for the cases of menoxenia or distending pain of the breast.

2. For cases with distending pain of the breast, add *Radix Salviae Miltiorrhizae* and *Fructus Hordei Germinatus* (30 g) to disperse the stagnated liver-qi and promote blood circulation; for cases with alternating epidsodes of chills and fever, omit *Ligustici Chuanxiong* and add *Radix Scutellariae* and *Herba Artemisiae Annuae* to clear away the gallbladder heat.

3. Also applicable to cases of pleurisy, cholecystitis, mastitis, hyperplasia of mammary gland, etc., which are attributive to stagnation of liver-qi and vital qi.

Decoction of Gentianae for Purging Liver-Fire
(Longdan xie gan tang)

Ingredients

Herba Gentianae	6 g
Radix Bupleuri	6 g
Radix Glycyrrhizae	6 g
Rhizoma Alismatis	10 g
Semen Plantaginis	10 g
Caulis Akebiae	10 g
Radix Rehmanniae	10 g
Fructus Gardeniae	10 g
Radix Scutellariae	10 g
Radix Angelicae Sinensis	3 g

Decoct the above ingredients in a right amount of water for oral administration.

Efficacy

.Purging the sthenia fire of liver and gallbladder, clearing away the dampness-heat evil from triple jiao; mainly for cases with flaming up of sthenia fire in the liver and gallbladder, manifested by headache, hypochondriac pain, bitter taste in the mouth, congestion of the conjunctiva and deafness, and for cases with downward attack of dampness-heat from the liver and gallbladder, manifested by stranguria with turbid urine, pruritus vulvae and leukorrhagia.

Indications

1. For cases of jaundice attributive to dampness-heat attacking the liver and gallbladder, omit *Glycyrrhizae* and *Rehmanniae* and add *Herba Artemisiae Scopariae* and *Radix et Rhizoma Rhei* to eliminate the heat evil through urination and defecation.

2. For cases of leukorrhagia, with yellow or red and white, thick, foul discharge, red tongue with yellowish and greasy fur, smooth and rapid pulse, which are attributive to downward attack of dampness-heat from the liver meridian, omit *Glycyrrhizae* and use *Cortex Phellodendri* instead of *Scutellariae*.

3. Also applicable to cases of acute conjunctivitis, acute otitis media, furuncle of the vestibulum nasi and external auditory canal, hypertension which are attributive to flaming up of sthenia fire in the liver and gallbladder; to cases of icteric hepatitis, cholecystitis, herpes zoster which are attributive to retention of dampness-heat evil in the liver and gallbladder; to cases of urinary infection, pelvic inflammation, prostatitis, which are attributive to downward attack of dampness-heat evil from the liver and gallbladder.

Pulse-Activating Powder
(Sheng mai san)

Ingredients

Radix Ginseng	10 g
Radix Ophiopogonis	15 g
Fructus Schisandrae	6 g

Decoct the above ingredients in a right amount of water for oral administration.

Efficacy

Supplementing qi, promoting the production of body fluid, astringing yin-fluid and arresting sweat.

Indications

Syndrome of impairment of both qi and yin manifested by general debility, shortness of breath, disinclination to talk, thirst with profuse sweat, dry tongue and throat, deficient and weak pulse, or impairment of the lung due to chronic cough, dry cough with shortness of breath, spontaneous perspiration or palpitation, and faint pulse with tendency to exhaustion.

The recipe can be modified to deal with dehydrant shock caused by heat stroke, bleeding, severe vomiting or diarrhea, dramatic injury, scald; or syndrome of impairment of both qi and yin as seen in cases at recovery stage of febrile diseases or at postoperation, or in cases with chronic disorders; or syndrome of deficiency of both qi and yin as seen in such cases as tuberculosis, chronic bronchitis, bronchiectasis, etc..

Cautions

Since it has an astringing effect, it is neither fit for patients whose exopathogen has not been dispelled, nor for those with hyperactivity of heat due to summer-heat diseases, but without impairment of qi and body fluid.

Decoction for Rashes Subsidence
(Hua ban tang)

Ingredients

Gypsum Fibrosum	30 g
Rhizoma Anemarrhenae	12 g
Radix Scrophulariae	10 g

Radix Glycyrrhizae	6 g
Cornu Rhinocerotis	6 g
Semen Oryzae Sativae	20 g

Decoct the above ingredients in a right amount of water for oral administration.

Efficacy

Clearing away heat evil and toxic material, cooling blood and letting tghe rashes subsided; mainly for cases attributive to involvement of qifen and xuefen by severe heat and extravasation of blood-heat, which are manifested by high fever, dark-red rashes, dry mouth, restlessness, or even unconsciousness and delinum, red tongue with yellow fur.

Indications

1. This prescription is applied for cases due to involvement of xuefen by severe heat in qifen, or involvement of both xuefen and qifen by severe heat.
2. Applicable to cases attributive to attack of the stomach by liver-fire with damage of the stomach vessels, which are manifested by hematemesis, irritability, red tongue with yellow fur, wiry and rapid pulse.
3. For cases attributive to hyperactivity of stomach-fire with involvement of blood, which are manifested by tooth bleeding, gingivitis, headache, foul breath, red tongue with yellow fur, bounding and rapid pulse, add *Radix Cyathulae* to let the fire running downward.
4. Also applicable to cses of typnus, erysipelas, epidemic meningitis, septicemia, etc. with fever and skin rashes attributive to involvement of qifen and xuefen by severe heat, or cases of esophageal varicosis with hematemesis attributive to attack of the stomach by liver-fire, or cases of periodontal diseases, necrotizing ulcerative gingivitis with tooth bleeding attributive to hyperactivity of stomach-fire.

Decoction of Restoration
(Fuyuan huoxue tang)

Ingredients

Radix Bupleuri	10 g
Radix Trichosanthis	10 g
Radix Angelicae Sinensis	10 g
Squama Manitis Praeparata	10 g
Radix et Rhizoma Rhei	10 g
Semen Persicae	10 g
Flos Carthami	6 g
Radix Glycyrrhizae	3 g
wine	q.s.

Decoct the above ingredients in a right amount of water for oral administration.

Efficacy

Activating blood circulation, removing blood stasis, dispersing the depressed liver-qi and dredging the passage of meridians; mainly for cases of swelling and pain over the chest and hypochondrium due to trauma.

Indications

1. This is a commonly-used prescription for traumata of chest and hypochondrium with swelling, pain and ecchymoses. For injury of the upper limbs, add *Ramulus Cinnamomi*; for that of the lower limbs, add *Radix Achyranthis Bidentatae*.

2. Also applicable to cases with chest intercostal neuralgia and costal chondritis which are attributive to retention of blood stasis.

Decoction for Severe Phlegm-Heat Syndrome in the Chest
(Da xian xiong tang)

Ingredients

Radix et Rhizoma Rhei	12 g
Natrii Sulfas	10 g
Radix Euphorbiae Kansui (powder, not for decocting)	1.5 g

Decoct the above ingredients in a right amount of water for oral administration.

Efficacy

Purging, eliminating water retention, relieving the accumulation of heat evil; mainly for syndrome attributive to evil accumulating in the thorax, manifested by severe pain and tenderness over the upper abdomen, fever, constipation, sunken and tense pulse, etc..

Indications

1. This prescription is applied for a critical case and should be used as early as possible. Diarrhea usually occurs half an hour after the decoction is taken. One dose may be repeated if diarrhea does not occur after one hour. Overdosage should be prohibited, otherwise the healthy qi may be impaired.

2. Also applicable to cases of acute pancreatitis edematous type, and acute cholecystitis, which are attributive to simultaneous attack of water and heat evil.

Decoction for Soothing the Intestine
(Chang ning tang)

Ingredients

Radix Angelicae Sinensis	15 g

Radix Rehmanniae Praeparata	15 g
Radix Codonopsis Pilosulae	10 g
Radix Ophiopogonis	10 g
Colla Corii Asini	10 g
Rhizoma Dioscoreae	10 g
Radix Dipsaci	10 g
Radix Glycyrrhizae	3 g
Cortex Cinnamomi	1 g

Decoct the above ingredients in a right amount of water for oral administration.

Efficacy

Nourishing blood and benefiting vital qi; mainly for cases of postpartum anemia with dull aching over the lower abdomen which can be relieved by pressing, discharge of scanty thin lochia, dizziness, tinnitus, palpitation, amnesia, pale complexion, constipation, pale tongue, small and weak pulse.

Indications

1. Applicable to cases of metrorrhagia with profuse thin and pale discharge, spiritlessness, dizziness, tinnitus, lumbago, weakness of knees, darkish complexion, pale tongue, sunken and small, weak pulse, which are attributive to impairment of liver and kidney and deficiency of blood and vital qi.

2. Also indicated for cases of ecthyma accompanied with pale tongue, small and rapid pulse, which are attributive to deficiency of blood and vital qi.

3. Also applicable to cases of chronic pelvic inflammation, hypofunction of anterior pituitary, chronic hypoadrenocorticism, dysfunctional uterine bleeding, phlebeurysma of lower limbs, chronic osteomyelitis, which are attributive to deficiency of blood and vital qi.

Decoction of Angelicae Sinensis for Analgesic
(Danggui niantong tang)

Ingredients

Rhizoma seu Radix Notopterygii	10 g
Herba Artemisiae Scopariae	10 g
Radix Ledebouriellae	10 g
Polyporus Umbellatus	10 g
Radix Puerariae	10 g
Rhizoma Atractylodis	10 g
Radix Angelicae Sinensis	12 g
Rhizoma Atractylodis Macrocephalae	12 g
Radix Scutellariae	8 g
Rhizoma Anemarrhenae	8 g
Rhizoma Alismatis	6 g
Rhizoma Cimicifugae	6 g
Radix Codonopsis Pilosulae	6 g
Radix Sophorae Flavescentis	6 g
Radix Glycyrrhizae Praeparata	3 g

Decoct the above ingredients in a right amount of water for oral administration.

Efficacy

Drying dampness, clearing away heat, activating blood circulation and expelling wind, mainly for cases attributive to attack of dampness and heat, which manifest swelling and pain of the joints, fever, aversion to wind, feeling of oppression over the chest, yellow and greasy fur on the tongue, soft and floating, slow or smooth and rapid pulse.

Indications

1. For cases of wet beriberi with oliguira, yellow and greasy fur on the

tongue, soft and floating, slow pulse, which are attributive to retention of dampness-heat in the meridians and stagnation of vital energy and blood, increase the dosage of *Atractylodis* and decrease the dose of *Scutellariae* and *Anemarrhenae*.

2. Also indicated for cases attributive to retention of dampness and toxic material in the muscles and skin, when manifest pyogenic infection of skin, accompanied with fever, thirst, yellow and greasy fur on tongue, soft and floating, slow pulse.

3. Also applicable to cases of rheumatic arthritis, periomarthritis, multiple neuritis, etc. which are attributive to retention of dampness-heat in the meridians; and to cases of impetigo, folliculitis, paronychia, etc. attributive to retention of dampness and toxic material in the muscles and skin.

Decoction of Angelicae Sinensis for Warming Cold Limbs
(Danggui sini tang)

Ingredients

Radix Angelicae Sinensis	10 g
Ramulus Cinnamomi	10 g
Radix Paeoniae Alba	12 g
Herba Asari	6 g
Radix Glycyrrhizae Praeparata	6 g
Caulis Akebiae	6 g
Fructus Ziziphi Jujubae	6 pcs

Decoct the above ingredients in a right amount of water for oral administration.

Efficacy

Warming the channel, expelling cold evil, nourishing blood and dredging the passage of channels; mainly for cases due to deficiency of blood, attack of cold evil and impediment of blood circulation, which are manifested by cold limbs, indistinct pulse, pale tongue with whitish fur.

Indications

1. For cases of dysmenorrhea attributive to deficiency of blood and presence of cold evil, omit *Akebiae* and add *Radix Rehmanniae Praeparata* to nourish the blood and regulate menstruation.

2. For cases with cold colic testalgia referring to the lower abdomen, sunken and wiry pulse, add *Fructus Foeniculi* to warm the liver and regulate vital energy.

4. Also aplicable to cases with cold limbs or abdominal pain occurring in thromboangiitis, *Raynaud's* disease, acrocyanosis, chilblain, indirect inguinal hernia, dysmenorrhea, etc., which are attributive to blood deficiency and affection of cold evil.

Decoction of Indigo Naturalis for Rashes Subsidence (Xiaoban qingdan san)

Ingredients

Indigo Naturalis	5 g
Rhizoma coptidis	12 g
Radix Scrophulariae	12 g
Cornu Rhinocerotis	9 g
Rhizoma Anemarrhenae	9 g
Fructus Gardeniae	9 g
Gypsum Fibrosum	30 g
Radix Codonopsis Pilosulae	6 g
Radix Bupleuri	6 g
Radix Glycyrrhizae	3 g
Rhizoma Zingiberis Recens	3 pcs
Fructus Ziziphi Jujubae	2 pcs
vinegar	a spoonful

Decoct the above ingredients in a right amount of water for oral administration.

Efficacy

Purging fire evil, eliminating toxic material, cooling blood and dispersing rashes; mainly for eruptive diseases of yang type attributive to hyperactivity of heat evil at both qifen and yingfen, and extravasation of blood, which are manifested by red rashes over the skin, high fever, irritability, thirst, red tongue with yellow and dry fur, bounding and smooth rapid pulse.

Indications

1. Applicable to cases of hematemesis with bright red or dark purplish bloody discharge, constipation or blackish stools, red tongue with yellow and dry fur, smooth and rapid pulse, which are attributive to damage of the stomach collateral by heat, and adverse rising of vital qi and fire.

2. For cases of burn manifested by local erythema, pain and heat, accompanied with high fever, irritability, thirst, constipation, red tongue with yellow and dry fur, bounding and rapid pulse, which are attributive to inward attack of potent fire evil and hyperactivity of heat at both qifen and yingfen, *Radix Ginseng* or *Radix panacis Quinquefolii* is used instead of *Codonopsis Pilosulae*.

3. Also applicable to cases of scarlet fever, dengue fever, typhus fever, erysipelas, exudative erythema multiforme, etc. with red eruptions and high fever, which are attributive to hyperactivity of heat at both qifen and yingfen, and extravasation of blood; also to cases of rupture of which are attributive to damage of stomach collateral by heat and adverse rising of vital qi and fire.

Decoction of Sargassum for Goiter
(Haizao yuhu tang)

Ingredients

Sargassum	9 g
Thallus Laminariae seu Eckloniae	9 g
Thallus Laminariae Japonicae	9 g
Rhizoma Pinelliae	9 g
Fructus Forsythiae	9 g
Bulbus Fritillariae Thunbergii	9 g
Radix Angelicae Sinensis	9 g
Radix Angelicae Pubescentis	6 g
Pericarpium Citri Reticulatae	6 g
Rhizoma Ligustici Chuanxiong	6 g
Exocarpium Citri Grandis	6 g
Radix Glycyrrhizae	3 g

Decoct the above ingredients in a right amount of water for oral administration.

Efficacy

Dispersing phlegm, softening masses, regulating qi and dispelling stagnation; mainly for goiter attributive to stagnation of phlegm and qi, which is round, soft, smooth and slowly growing, with wiry pulse.

Indications

1. For scrofula attributive to stagnation of phlegm and vital qi, which are hard and movable, accompanied with wiry and smooth pulse, omit *Angelicae Pubescentis* from the prescription.

2. Indicated for hard, movable and slow-growing masses of the breast, accompanied with wiry pulse, which are attributive to the stagnation of phlegm and vital qi.

3. Also applicable to adenoma of thyroid, nodular goiter, thyroiditis, cervical lymphadenitis, fibrodenoma and cystic hyperplasia of the breast.

Pill for Eliminating Phlegm Evil
(Gun Tan Wan)

Ingredients

Radix et Rhizoma Rhei	240 g
Radix Scutellariae	240 g
Lignum Aquilariae Resinatum	15 g
Lapis Chloriti	30 g

Efficacy

Purging fire and eliminating phlegm; mainly for cases of chronic phlegm-syndrome of sthenic heat type, manifested by mania with frigtening, or dyspneic cough with thick sputum, or feeling of oppression over the chest and epigastrium, or dizziness with profuse expectoration, constipationm, yellow and thick, greasy fur on the tongue, smooth and rapid, strong pulse.

Indications

1. This formula cannot be taken as decoction.
2. Applicable to cases of nasosinusitis manifested by stuffy nose, headache, turbid, foul, thick and yellow nasal discharge, yellow and greasy fur on the tongue, wiry and rapid pulse, which are attributive to the attack of phlegm-heat from the spleen and stomach to the nasal orifice.

3. Applicable to cases of chronic suppurative otitis media accompanied with deafness, tinnitus, yellow and greasy fur on the tongue, wiry and rapid pulse, which are attributive to the attack of dampness-heat of lvier and gallbladder to the orifice.

4. Applicable to cases of schizophrenia, manic-depressive psychosis, chronic bronchitis, emphysema, etc., which are attributive to chronic phlegm-syndrome of sthenic heat type.

图书在版编目(CIP)数据

中医美容:英文版/赵昕,李国华主编-北京:学苑出版社,1998.2
ISBN7-5077-0358-4

Ⅰ.中… Ⅱ.①赵… ②李… Ⅲ.①中医-美容-方法-英文 Ⅳ.TS974

中国版本图书馆 CIP 数据核字(98)第 00905 号

中医美容

主编 赵 昕 李国华

学苑出版社出版
(中国北京万寿路西街 11 号)
邮政编码 100036
北京大兴沙窝店印刷厂印刷
中国国际图书贸易总公司发行
(中国北京车公庄西路 35 号)
北京邮政信箱第 399 号 邮政编码 100044
英文版 16 开本
1998 年 2 月第 1 版第 1 次印刷
ISBN7-5077-0358-4

06850
14-E-2920P